Alloimmunity:
1993 and Beyond

Alloimmunity: 1993 and Beyond

Editor

Sandra Taddie Nance, MS, MT(ASCP)SBB
Assistant Director, Technical Services
American Red Cross Blood Services
Penn-Jersey Region
Philadelphia, Pennsylvania

American Association of Blood Banks
Bethesda, Maryland
1993

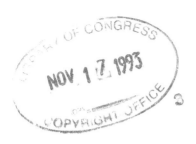

American Association of Blood Banks   ISBN NO. 1-56395-025-1
8101 Glenbrook Road   Printed in the United States
Bethesda, Maryland 20814-2749

Library of Congress Cataloging-in-Publication Data

Alloimmunity— 1993 and beyond / editor, Sandra Taddie Nance.
p. cm.
Includes bibliographical references and index.
ISBN 1-56395-025-1
1. Immunohematology. 2. Blood—Transfusion—Complications.
I. Nance, Sandra Taddie. II. American Association of Blood Banks.
RB45.5.A45 1993
616.07'9—dc20
93-32964
CIP

 Text paper meets EPA guidelines for minimum recovered material content
(50% recycled fiber, including 10% postconsumer waste)

Scientific Program Committee

Sandra Taddie Nance, MS, MT(ASCP)SBB
Chairman

Richard H. Aster, MD
Michael P. Busch, MD, PhD
Roger Y. Dodd, PhD
Jay Epstein, MD
Dennis Goldfinger, MD
Gregory R. Halverson, MT(ASCP)SBB
Peter D. Issitt, PhD, FIMLS, FIBiol, FRCPath
Steven H. Kleinman, MD
Naomi L.C. Luban, MD
Leslie E. Silberstein, MD
Marilyn J. Telen, MD
Patricia Tippett, PhD

Contents

Foreword

This year's Annual Seminar Book contains chapters by eminent transfusion medicine scientists and is titled "Alloimmunity: 1993 and Beyond." The focal point of the book is the fourth chapter written by the 1993 Emily Cooley Lecturer, Richard H. Aster, MD. His chapter, "Platelet-Specific Alloantigen Systems: History, Clinical Significance and Molecular Biology," with over 150 references, is an excellent chapter that assimilates most of what is known about the field.

The book begins with a chapter by Glenn E. Rodey, MD (Atlanta, GA) on "Cellular Immune Responses to Alloimmunization." This chapter reviews immunologic recognition of antigens and the cellular elements of an immune response, including antigen-presenting cells, dendritic cells, B lymphocytes and macrophages. Further topics include HLA molecules in antigen presentation, B lymphocytes and T lymphocytes. A portion of the chapter details the special circumstances of alloimmunization, including self-reactivity, size of the alloreactive T-cell repertoire, allorecognition pathways and donor dendritic cells in allorecognition. Of particular value for teaching purposes are the figures giving schematic representations of cellular interactions.

The second chapter, "The Antibody Response to Antigen," is written by Leslie E. Silberstein, MD (Philadelphia, PA). This chapter continues to expand our knowledge of alloimmunity, first discussing the humoral immune response, then features of antibody responses. Part of the chapter covers antibody diversity at the serologic level and the genetic basis for antibody diversity. Dr. Silberstein's writings take the reader from the very simple to the very complex quite easily. Monoclonal, pathologic anti-I/i cold agglutinins are discussed as well as clinically insignificant anti-I/i. This chapter also contains some elegant figures that show schematics of phases of humoral response, B-cell differentiation, proliferation and antibody secretion, role of cytokines, T-cell-independent and T-cell and B-cell collaboration.

The third chapter, written by Jeffrey McCullough, MD; Mary E. Clay, MS, MT(ASCP); and David F. Stroncek, MD (St. Paul, MI), is titled "Granulocyte Alloantigen Systems and Their Clinical Significance." The chapter is an excellent review of the alloantigen systems of granulocytes. The biochemistry of the granulocyte-specific antigens and the molecules of the granulocyte membrane are discussed. The relationship of granulocyte antigens to other granulocyte membrane molecules is covered. Another section describes clinical situations involving alloantibodies of the granulocyte system.

As noted earlier, the fourth chapter is written by the 1993 Emily Cooley lecturer, Richard H. Aster, MD (Milwaukee, WI). This comprehensive chapter highlights posttransfusion purpura and neonatal alloimmune thrombocytopenia. The molecular basis of platelet-specific alloantigens is detailed and marvelous figures are provided to clarify what is known about the antigens. Dr. Aster also discusses the immune response to platelet specific alloantigens.

The next chapter, "New and Evolving Techniques for Antibody and Antigen Identification," was written by Marilyn J. Telen, MD (Durham, NC). The chapter describes the concept of antigens as epitopes and genetically engineered blood group antigen expression. Antigen systems about which relatively more is known at the molecular level are discussed. Dr. Telen gives us a look into the future of immunohematologic testing.

The sixth chapter, "New Insights Into the Pathophysiology and Treatment of Acute Hemolytic Transfusion Reactions," was written by Stephen M. Capon, MD (San Diego, CA) and Dennis Goldfinger, MD (Los Angeles, CA). The classification, immunology and pathophysiology are reviewed from the perspective of traditional concepts. The recently reported role of cytokines in hemolytic transfusion reactions is highlighted, with particular emphasis on how this may influence treatment.

"Prenatal and Perinatal Management of Alloimmune Cytopenias," the seventh chapter, was written by Janice G. McFarland, MD (Milwaukee, WI). The focus of this chapter is on clinical management of hemolytic disease of the newborn and fetus and neonatal and fetal alloimmune thrombocytopenia. The pathophysiology, clinical features, antenatal management and neonatal management are discussed for each of these results of maternal alloimmunization.

The final chapter, "Prospects for Modulation of Alloimmunity," was written by David D. Eckels, PhD (Milwaukee, WI). The chapter presents the phenomena of alloimmunity, the various molecular structures involved, the consequences of alloimmune recognition and, lastly, the ways in which alloimmunity might be modulated.

This book, *Alloimmunity: 1993 and Beyond*, provides the reader with eight different topics on alloimmunity. This book will prove to be useful to transfusion medicine specialists as well as students by providing comprehensive reviews and references that are current as of May 1993. The Scientific Program Committee of the American Association of Blood Banks enthusiastically recommends this timely book.

Sandra Taddie Nance, MS, MT(ASCP)SBB
Editor

The Emily Cooley Lecture

Today's lecture is the 30th in a series of annual lectures in honor of Emily Cooley, an outstanding medical technologist.

Emily Cooley was an attractive young woman raised in a distinguished family—her grandfather had been a Justice of the Supreme Court of Michigan and her father was a professor of pediatrics at Wayne State University. She had been brought up to be an artist, or a writer, or simply to preside over a household like her mother. She had attended a private school for girls and graduated from Vassar College with a degree in landscaping. Her mother, a kindly, gracious woman, was often incapacitated with attacks of melancholia and her father, then about to retire, was ailing much of the time. Emily ran the household and was her father's companion, chauffeur, travel aide, nurse, secretary and illustrator. It was she who drew the beautiful illustrations of blood films that appeared in Dr. Cooley's publications.

After the death of both her parents, Emily had to find a career in which to earn a living. Having been so intimately connected with medicine, and hematology in particular, she chose medical technology. She took her training at Henry Ford Hospital and received a master's degree before she started work. Returning to Children's Hospital, where her father had worked in the laboratory, she became the chief hematology technologist. An excellent morphologist, Emily became the mainstay of her department and was looked up to and beloved by her colleagues.

Emily Cooley was not only a fine technologist and a dedicated worker in the laboratory but also a warm, sensitive, intelligent and gracious human being. It is to her memory that this series of lectures is dedicated.

Emily Cooley Lecturers

1963 .... E. Eric Muirhead, MD
1964 .... Scott N. Swisher, MD
1965 .... Wolf W. Zuelzer, MD
1966 .... Alexander S. Wiener, MD
1967 .... Max M. Strumia, MD
1968 .... Hugh Chaplin, Jr., MD
1969 .... Emanuel Hackel, PhD
1970 .... Flemming Kissmeyer-Nielsen, MD, PhD
1971 .... Neva Martin Abelson, MD
1972 .... Bernard Pirofsky, MD
1973 .... Serafeim P. Masouredis, MD, PhD
1974 .... Paul J. Schmidt, MD
1975 .... Eloise R. Giblett, MD
1976 .... Richard E. Rosenfield, MD
1977 .... Herbert F. Polesky, MD
1978 .... Mary N. Crawford, MD
1979 .... Sir John Dacie, MD, FRCP, FRCPath, FRS
1980 .... Kathryn M. Beattie, MT(ASCP)SBB
1981 .... C. Paul Engelfriet, MD
1982 .... Edwin A. Steane, PhD
1983 .... Marjory Stroup, MT(ASCP)SBB
1984 .... Patrick L. Mollison, CBE, MD, FRCP,
                              FRCPath, FRCOG, FRS
1985 .... Jeffrey McCullough, MD
1986 .... Peter D. Issitt, PhD, FIMLS, FIBiol, FRCPath
1987 .... Harvey J. Alter, MD
1988 .... W. Laurence Marsh, PhD, FRCPath, FIBiol,
                              FIMLS
1989 .... George Garratty, PhD, FIMLS, MRCPath
1990 .... Sherrill J. Slichter, MD
1991 .... Lawrence D. Petz, MD
1992 .... Herbert A. Perkins, MD

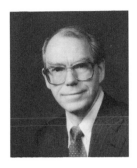

1993 Emily Cooley
Memorial Lecturer:

Richard H. Aster, MD

Richard H. Aster, MD, will present the 1993 Emily Cooley Memorial Lecture. Dr. Aster earned his MD from the University of Michigan Medical School and did his internship and residency at the Massachusetts General Hospital. He was a Clinical Associate in Hematology at the National Institutes of Health (NIH) and took a fellowship in hematology on the Harvard Medical Service of the Boston City Hospital. He served as an Instructor, Associate, and Assistant Professor of Medicine at the Harvard Medical School, prior to relocating to Milwaukee, where he is President of The Blood Center of Southeastern Wisconsin and Clinical Professor of Medicine and Pathology at the Medical College of Wisconsin.

Dr. Aster has been the recipient of many awards. He was a Regents-Alumni Scholar as an undergraduate at the University of Michigan and the recipient of a special scholarship at the University of Michigan Medical School. He received a Research Career Development Award and a MERIT Award from the National Heart, Lung, and Blood Institute as well as two distinguished Service Awards, one from the Milwaukee Academy of Medicine and the second from the Medical College of Wisconsin.

Dr. Aster is an active member of 19 professional societies and has served on committees and/or boards of directors of most of them. We are particularly fortunate that one of the 19 is the American Association of Blood Banks where he has served on the Committees on Standards, Scientific Program and Scientific Advisory Committees and is an Associate Editor of our journal, *Transfusion*.

Dr. Aster is married and is the father of five sons. The oldest is pursuing a medical career and the youngest is in high school. His outside interests include golf, tennis and travel. He hopes to be able to allocate more time to those pursuits at some point in the future.

The American Association of Blood Banks is proud to award the 1993 Emily Cooley Memorial Award to Dr. Richard H. Aster, a world-renowned researcher and educator who has authored more than 234 full-length publications.

In: Nance ST, ed.
Alloimmunity: 1993 and Beyond
Bethesda, MD: American Association of Blood Banks, 1993

1

Cellular Immune Responses to Alloimmunization

Glenn E. Rodey, MD

A LLOIMMUNIZATION MAY OCCUR WHEN cells or tissues of one individual are transferred to a second individual of the same species through pregnancy, blood transfusion or tissue transplantation. Any foreign allelic molecules, including red cell antigens, immunoglobulins, platelet-specific antigens or major histocompatibility complex (MHC) gene products, potentially can induce alloimmunization.

Immune responses historically have been divided into antibody-mediated and cell-mediated immune responses, depending upon whether final effector mechanisms are mediated by B-cell products or by T cells. This simple division, however, misrepresents the complexity of cellular interactions that culminate in an immune response. For example, specific antibody production by B cells to most protein antigens does not occur unless T-helper cells first activate B cells. Further, exposure to an immunogen under circumstances in which critical cell-mediated costimulatory signals are not delivered leads to anergy of T cells rather than to their activation into effector immune responses.

In this chapter, cellular responses that occur during primary alloimmunization, broadly defined as the functional interactions of antigen-presenting cells, T cells and B cells, will be reviewed. Discussions will focus on alloimmunity to human HLA gene products, since these responses play a dominant role in platelet transfusion, solid organ and bone marrow transplantation outcomes. To facilitate discussion of the complex cellular interactions involved in alloimmunization, a brief review of the general features of an immune response and the functional attributes of individual cellular elements in an immune response is first presented.

Glenn E. Rodey, MD, Professor, Department of Pathology, Emory University School of Medicine, Atlanta, Georgia

Immunologic Recognition of Antigens

Antigen-specific recognition of foreign antigens by the adaptive immune system is governed by three genetic systems: 1) Class I and Class II MHC genes, 2) T-cell receptor genes and 3) B-cell receptor (immunoglobulin) genes. B cells, through their membrane immunoglobulin (MIg) receptors, can interact directly with epitope conformations present on native, unmodified antigens such as foreign HLA molecules or hepatitis B surface antigen. In contrast to B-cell receptors, antigen-specific T-cell receptors (TCRs) recognize a heterodimeric complex consisting of an antigen-derived peptide that is noncovalently bound to an HLA molecule.[1,2]

Engagement of the specific antigen receptors of B or T cells by the appropriate ligands during a primary response is insufficient to activate a B cell to produce antibody, or a T cell to synthesize cytokines or acquire the function of cytotoxicity. Additional signals must be received by both cell types before activation can occur. In fact, there is abundant evidence that engagement of antigen receptors in the absence of critical costimulatory signals can deactivate cells and may prevent their activation by subsequent exposure to antigen (anergy).[3-5] For B cells with receptors specific for protein antigens, the additional signals are provided primarily by T-helper cells. This response is referred to as a T-dependent B-cell response.[6-11] For T-cell responses, the signals are provided by antigen-presenting cells, which may be dendritic cells in a primary response and, additionally, B cells, or macrophages in a secondary response.[12-14]

The mechanisms required to get target antigens, antigen-presenting cells, T cells and B cells together effectively, in vivo, eluded immunologists for many years. Some of these mysteries have been clarified through better understanding of lymph node, spleen and other peripheral lymphoid tissue physiology, and through the recognition of several families of membrane-associated adhesion molecules. These specialized molecules are the road signs by which lymphocytes move and traffic throughout the body, and they provide the essential language of cell-to-cell communications in the immune system. Naive T and B cells recirculate through defined pathways that include the blood, afferent lymphatic channels, specific regions in the organized secondary lymphoid tissues, and efferent lymphatic channels. Circulation continues until the cells die or encounter an appropriate antigen or signal. Antigen-activated and memory T cells develop additional adhesion molecules that permit egress from capillaries and into sites of inflammation, where they may then be retained by other specific adhesion molecules. Collectively, distribution of adhesion molecules on various T and B cell subpopulations defines precise and distinct homing routes. These molecules interact with complementary ligands present on endothelial cells and various extracellular matrices. The role of adhesion molecules in lymphocyte trafficking was recently reviewed.[15]

Similar receptor-ligand interactions allow T cells to transiently engage antigen-presenting cells and other T or B cells in "conversation." If nothing important is learned, that is, the T-cell antigen receptor is not engaged, the cells dissociate and the T cell interacts with the next cell it contacts.[11,16] CD4 and CD8 molecules may transiently interact with Class II and I molecules during this process. Representative examples of receptors and counter receptors are shown in Table 1-1.

Cellular Elements of an Immune Response

Antigen-Presenting Cells (APCs)

The term "antigen-presenting cell" refers to a set of functional attributes of different cell types that permit them to effectively present

Table 1-1. Examples of Adhesion or Other Interactive Molecules on Lymphocytes and Dendritic Cells

Molecule	Ligand	T Cells	B Cells	Dendritic Cells
TCR	MHC/peptide	+		
MIg	Antigen		+	
CD4/CD8	MHC I or II	+		
FcR	Ig	+/−	+	
B7	CD28		+*	+*
CD28	B7	+		
CD40	B-cell AF†		+	+
B-cell AF†	CD40	+		
CD2	LFA-3	+		
LFA-3	CD2			+
LFA-1	ICAMs	+	+	
ICAMs	LFA-1			+
CD11c	C‡			+
IL2-R	IL-2	+		+
β1-integrins	ECM§	+		
CD22	CD45RO	+		
CD45RO	CD22	+		

*Expressed on activated cells
†B-cell activating factor present in the membrane of activated T cells
‡Complement
§Extracellular matrices such as fibronectin, vitronectin, collagen, lominin

peptides to T cells. During a primary immune response, the major cell type that can perform this function for naive, resting T cells is the dendritic cell.[17-19] B lymphocytes and, to a lesser extent, macrophages can also present antigen to memory T cells previously exposed to the inducing antigen.[20] Effective activation of antigen-specific T cells by APCs involves four steps: 1) uptake and partial degradation of the antigen into peptides that bind to intracellular MHC molecules (processing), 2) re-expression of the peptide-MHC molecules on the cell membrane surface (presentation), 3) interaction of the T-cell antigen receptor with the peptide-MHC complex and 4) interaction of accessory receptors with their ligands.

Dendritic Cells

Dendritic cells are derived from hematopoietic stem cells and at some point during differentiation develop into a specific lineage of cells distinct from monocytes and macrophages.[19,21] They are widely distributed in small numbers throughout most organs in the body and are especially numerous within the skin (Langerhans cells), mucous membrane barriers of the gastrointestinal and respiratory tracts and portal triads of the liver. Although they comprise less than 0.1% of peripheral blood leukocytes, they are the major stimulator cell in mixed leukocyte cultures.[18] Special attributes of dendritic cells include a high density of membrane Class I and II molecules, a transient capacity for endocytosis and the ability to generate additional co-stimulatory signals required for activation of resting T cells whose antigen receptors have engaged MHC/peptide heterodimers.

In-vivo dendritic cells have several functional properties that make them well-suited to deliver antigen to small numbers of antigen-specific T cells. In peripheral tissues, they serve as sentinels, capturing foreign antigens by unknown mechanisms. The process of antigen capture appears to upregulate the expression of surface HLA Class I and II molecules and to induce endocytosis, antigen processing and antigen presentation on HLA molecules.[22] Within hours of antigen capture, dendritic cells become mobile and migrate through blood or afferent lymphatic channels to T-cell regions of the spleen or regional lymph nodes. This migratory process brings the processed antigen to the site through which circulating T cells pass, increasing the odds that antigen-specific T cells will encounter the relevant antigen. Once contact occurs between the dendritic cell and antigen-specific T cells, stable clusters are formed and T-cell activation proceeds. Owing to their large surface area, dendritic cells can bind as many as 10-20 lymphocytes.[23] Costimulatory signals provided by dendritic cells are still poorly characterized, but they require direct cell contact.[24] B7, a ligand for CD28 expressed on T cells, is upregulated in activated Langerhans cells, and is a major candidate for costimulatory function.

In a primary humoral response, naive antigen-specific B cells are thought to interact with dendritic cell T-cell clusters in T-cell zones (Fig 1-1), initiating B-cell activation, proliferation and immunoglobulin synthesis.[25]

B Lymphocytes and Macrophages

B cells and macrophages can process and present antigen to memory T cells,[9] but both are relatively ineffective in antigen presentation to naive, resting T cells. Although the spectrum of costimulatory signals required in different cellular interactions is still poorly characterized, more than one set of receptor-ligand interaction is probably necessary for each cell-to-cell interaction. B cells or macrophages may present

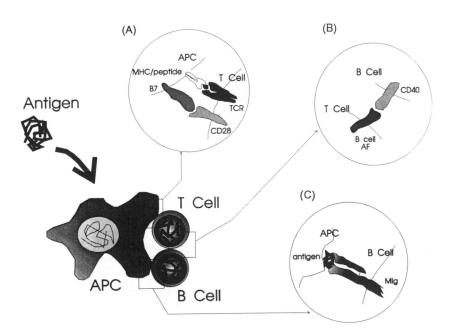

Figure 1-1. Summary of the major receptor/ligand interactions that occur during a primary humoral immune response. Antigen-specific and co-stimulator interactions are enlarged. In (A), (APC-T-cell interaction), the T-cell receptor binds to the MHC Class II/peptide complex. B7 and CD28 interact to provide a costimulatory signal. In (B), (T-cell-B-cell interaction), T cells activate B cells through binding of membrane-bound B activating factor (AF) with the B-cell ligand, CD40. In (C), (APC-B cell interaction), the B-cell receptor (MIg) binds to native antigen on the surface of the APC. APC = antigen-presenting cell.

antigen effectively to memory T cells because certain costimulatory signals provided by dendritic cells during a primary T-cell response may not be required for activation of memory T cells.[26] Thus, memory T cells potentially may be activated by cells expressing Class II molecules containing relevant peptides other than recognized antigen-presenting cells. This mode of T-cell activation may account for the persistence of certain autoimmune diseases or of chronic allograft rejection. In both settings, Class II molecules are often induced on cells, through the action of proinflammatory cytokines such as interferon gamma, that normally do not express these molecules constitutively.[27]

B lymphocytes are especially efficient antigen-presenting cells to memory T cells because of the presence of antigen-specific MIg. Antigen bound to MIg is internalized through receptor-mediated endocytosis, is processed, and immunogenic peptides are re-expressed in association with Class II MHC molecules. Receptor-mediated endocytosis is approximately 1000 times more efficient in capturing specific antigens and processing peptides than the random endocytosis of antigen by macrophages.[28(p 8.13)] The other essential costimulatory factor for T-cell antigen presentation, B7 molecule expression, is induced on B cells following their activation.

The primary function of the macrophage exposed to antigen is complete antigen degradation and disposal through lysosomal compartments. However, a small quantity of antigen is also processed in acidic endosomal compartments and presented on MHC molecules to T cells. As noted, antigen presentation by these cells is of relatively low efficiency compared with either dendritic cells or B cells.

HLA Molecules in Antigen Presentation

Involvement of HLA molecules in antigen presentation was observed in the early 1970's by Zinkernagel and Doherty.[1] Cytotoxic T lymphocytes (CTLs) generated against specific virus-infected cells only killed virus-infected cells bearing MHC antigens shared by the original infected stimulator cell. This phenomenon is referred to as MHC-restricted responses. Bjorkman and colleagues determined the three-dimensional structure of the HLA-A2 Class I molecule in 1987[2,29] and provided a structural basis for the presentation of peptides by HLA molecules. HLA Class I and, by deduction, HLA Class II molecules[30] bear a pocket formed by the two membrane-distal domains of the molecule (Fig 1-2). This "peptide groove" serves as a binding site for a variety of peptides. The T-cell antigen receptor thus interacts directly with both peptide and MHC molecule (Fig 1-3).

Peptides presented by MHC molecules are derived from two distinct sources: 1) exogenously derived antigens that are taken into cells and ultimately presented on Class II MHC molecules to CD4-positive T cells[31] (this is the classical pathway utilized by antigen-presenting

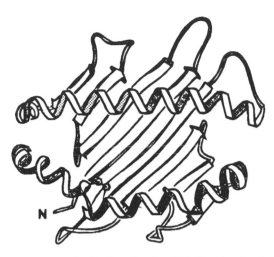

Figure 1-2. Schematic of the peptide binding site of an HLA Class I molecule (HLA-A2), viewed from the perspective of a T-cell receptor. The groove that binds peptides consists of a floor formed by beta-pleated sheets and two walls formed by alpha helices. In Class I molecules, the peptide binding site is derived from the alpha-1 and alpha-2 domains of the heavy chain. In Class II molecules, the structure is formed from the alpha-1 and beta-1 domains of the alpha and beta chains. (Used with permission from Bjorkman et al.[2])

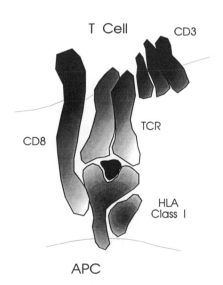

Figure 1-3. A schematic illustration of the T-cell receptor and CD8 molecules interacting with the MHC Class I/peptide complex. The T-cell receptor complex (TCR and CD3) recognizes and binds to a configuration formed by the Class I MHC molecule and its specific bound peptide (shown in black). The CD8 molecule of the T cell also binds to a site in the alpha-3 domain of the Class I molecule, increasing the binding strength of the interaction and providing additional costimulatory signals.

cells to capture, process and present antigens for subsequent induction of delayed type hypersensitivity reactions or the production of antibodies) and 2) endogenous antigens that originate in the cytosolic internal environment of the cell.[32] Endogenous peptides, which may include peptides from self antigens or may be derived from early viral proteins produced in a virus-infected cell, are presented primarily by Class I MHC molecules and are recognized by CD8-positive CTLs. The routes through which the peptides and the Class II or I molecules pass are referred to respectively as the exogenous and endogenous pathways, according to the origin of the peptides (Fig 1-4).

Exogenous Pathway

With appropriate route of administration, foreign antigen derived from the external environment is taken up by APCs via random or receptor-mediated endocytosis. The antigen undergoes limited proteolysis within membrane-bound endosomal compartments. Concurrently, MHC Class II molecules are assembled in the endoplasmic reticulum. Early Class II molecules contain a third chain, in addition to the alpha and beta, called the invariant or gamma chain. The chain serves two important functions in the exogenous pathway: 1) it occupies the peptide binding groove and prevents most endogenously derived peptides from binding to the newly assembled Class II molecules and 2) it contains an amino acid sequence that targets the molecule to the endosomal compartments (confusingly called the endocytic route). Upon entry into endosomes, the invariant chain is degraded, freeing the peptide groove to bind newly formed peptides that were specifically derived from exogenous antigens. The peptide/MHC complex is then transported to the plasma membrane and is re-expressed on its surface. The peptide groove of Class II molecules appears to be open on one side and can accommodate peptides of variable length, usually about 13-17 amino acids in length.[34] By contrast, both ends of the Class I peptide groove are closed, restricting the size of peptides that can be accommodated to 8-10 amino acids in length.[35]

Endogenous Pathway

Peptides presented by Class I MHC molecules have their origins mainly from proteins found in the cytosol. A majority of them are derived from self proteins under normal circumstances. Endogenous peptides are also derived from viral proteins when these proteins are actively synthesized by a virus-infected cell.[36] Recent evidence indicates that peptides from phagocytosed microbial antigens also can gain access to newly synthesized Class I molecules via novel and undefined mechanisms.[37] It appears that evolution has provided the

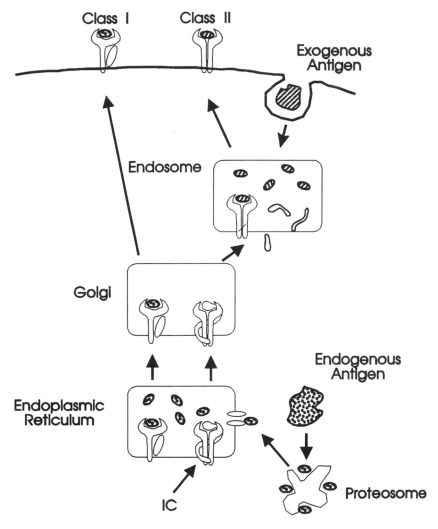

Figure 1-4. Scheme demonstrating the endogenous (stippled antigen) and exogenous (striped antigen) pathways of antigen presentation. Exogenous antigens are partially digested in endosomal compartments. Class II molecules, whose peptide binding sites are occupied by an invariant chain (IC), traffic to the endosomal compartment, where the IC is degraded. The exogenous peptides are then loaded into the peptide binding sites and the complexes are transported to and expressed on the cell membrane. Endogenously derived antigens originating in the cytosol are partially degraded by proteosomal bodies, then actively transported into the endoplasmic reticulum. Here, they bind with the Class I molecules, forming stable complexes that enter the Golgi apparatus and are transported directly to the cell membrane. (Modified with permission from Long EO.[33])

endogenous pathway and Class I MHC molecules as a mechanism to survey the internal environment of the cell for antigens from replicating organs and from mutated self proteins that would otherwise escape recognition by antibody or other extracellular immune mechanisms. In contrast to Class II molecules, whose structure is temporarily stabilized by the invariant chain prior to peptide binding in endosomal compartments, Class I molecules must bind peptides within the endoplasmic reticulum. Otherwise, the association of the Class I heavy chain with beta-2-microglobulin is highly unstable.[36,38,39] Cytosolic antigens appear to be degraded into a series of short peptides through the action of proteosome-like bodies, although the requirement for the MHC-linked proteosomal units in peptide presentation to Class I molecules has recently been questioned.[40,41] These peptides, which are transported into the endoplasmic reticulum by transporter proteins, specifically bind with the assembling Class I molecules to produce stable trimeric complexes. Finally, the complexes are transported directly to the plasma membrane and re-expressed on the membrane surface.

B Lymphocytes and Antibody

B cells and humoral immunity will be discussed in detail in Chapter 2. However, antibody production is a major component of the immune response to alloimmunization, and a small summary of the cellular events preceding antibody production is warranted. Although B cells can directly respond to certain carbohydrate antigens containing repetitive epitopes that crosslink MIg receptors, the majority of responses require a signal provided by T-helper cells. As noted, both naive T and B cells recirculate; and a primary immune response usually occurs in T-cell zones of secondary lymphoid tissues. It is generally recognized that efficient antibody production by B cells involves cognate interaction with T cells having specificity for the same antigen.[9] This close relationship can easily be visualized in a secondary response in which antigen-specific B cells directly process and present antigen to T cells. It is more difficult to envision this process in a primary response, since dendritic cells must present antigen to T cells; therefore, a three-cell interaction must be required for specific antibody production, but the exact mechanisms are not clear. Three-cell cognate interactions might be feasible if we assume that, in addition to processed antigen, the dendritic cell may also carry elements of native antigen on its surface.[42] In this setting, naive B cells and T cells would independently recognize and interact with antigen-laden dendritic cells—B cells recognizing native antigen and T cells recognizing processed antigen presented on Class II molecules. The T cell would undergo activation, and antigen-specific B cells, in close proximity to the activated T cells, would be positioned to receive the

T-cell signal necessary for their activation. The profile of lymphokines secreted by the T cell during the activation process dictates the type of heavy chain class switching the B cell will undergo. At a later stage, activated B cells migrate into primary follicles and undergo clonal expansion and immunoglobulin gene somatic mutations, leading to the production of high affinity antibody-producing cells and memory B cells.[25] Antigen, in the form of antigen-antibody complexes, can be retained in germinal centers for months or years, providing an ongoing source of antigen to sustain populations of memory B cells.[42] Increasing evidence indicates that memory B cells eventually undergo apoptosis and death if antigen or other rescue signals are not provided to the cells on a regular basis.[43,44] Thus, sustained antibody titers in a highly sensitized individual imply the persistence of an antigen source or an anti-idiotypic antibody bearing an internal image of the antigen.

Defined mechanisms of crosstalk between B and memory T cells are gradually emerging. Activated T cells develop membrane-associated B-cell activating molecules that interact with a constitutively expressed B-cell receptor termed CD40.[45] This interaction activates the B cell and causes it to proliferate. B7, the activation molecule induced on dendritic cells following their activation, is also expressed constitutively on monocytes, macrophages and activated B cells. Each of these cell types can present antigen to T cells and can influence the profiles of cytokines synthesized by the activated T cell. Recently, Galvin and colleagues[14] transfected genes for B7 and an intact MHC Class II molecule into Chinese hamster ovary (CHO) cells and demonstrated effective in-vitro presentation of ovalbumin to T cells from previously immunized mice. Thus, the combination of B7 and MHC/peptide complex appears to permit efficient presentation to memory T cells.

T Lymphocytes

T cells have emerged as essential elements in virtually every form of immune response. Two general phenotypic categories of T cells, CD4 positive and CD8 positive, have been known for over a decade. The division, which broadly defined functional categories of cells having the general properties of helper/inducer cells and cytotoxic/suppressor cells, spurred rapid growth in the discipline of cellular immunology. With time, it became apparent that the functions of these two populations were not always mutually exclusive. In 1986, Mosmann[46,47] and subsequently others[48-51] observed that both of these phenotypic cell types could be further subdivided into discrete functional categories according to the profile of lymphokines they secrete. This seminal observation has created a second major conceptual growth phase in cellular immunology.

Th1 and Th2 Subsets

Mice, rats and humans can develop, during the course of an immune response, T-helper populations having distinct cytokine profiles (Table 1-2). One type, referred to as Th1, secretes predominantly IL-2 and IFN-γ. Upon activation, Th1 cells express IL-2 receptors and use this lymphokine as an autocrine growth factor. These cytokine profiles play a major role in the mediation of delayed-type sensitivity (DTH) reactions and are dominantly found in chronic inflammatory lesions classically mediated by DTH. Th1 cells are capable of activating B cells and causing their proliferation, but the cytokine profile secreted by these cells does not induce significant heavy chain class switching in B cells.[52,53]

In contrast, a second type, referred to as Th2, secretes predominantly IL-4, IL-5 and IL-10. Th2 cells express IL-4 receptors and can use this cytokine as an autocrine receptor.[54] Cytokines produced by Th2 are essential for heavy chain switching in activated B cells to G, A or E class immunoglobulin production. Th2 cells are the principal T-helper cells for B-cell maturation and antibody production.[52,53] Th2 cells are also predominantly found in chronic inflammatory lesions in which IgE, mast cells and eosinophils are major effector mechanisms, such as atopic allergic reactions and parasitic infestations.

Not all CD4-positive, T-helper cells show the distinctive cytokine profiles of Th1 and Th2 cells. In fact, a commonly observed profile in humans is T cells (called Th0) that produce most of the cytokines produced by both Th1 and Th2. Th0 cells may represent activated T cells not yet committed to a discrete pathway of cytokine synthesis. The various T-cell subsets may not be distinct lineages (see below), but, rather, cells that have received different, activating signals.[46] Some evidence indicates that CD8-positive

Table 1-2. Differences in the Profile of Lymphokines Secreted by Human T-Helper Subsets[47]

Lymphokine	CD4 Positive	
	Th1	Th2
IL-2	+ +	+
IFN-γ	+ +	−
IL-4	−	+ +
IL-5	−	+ +
IL-10	+ /−	+ +
TNF-α	+ +	+
GM-CSF	+ +	+ +

T cells similarly may be divided into populations with Th1- and Th2-like cytokine profiles.[50]

Regulation of Th1 and Th2 Subsets

Th1 and Th2 cells are mutually regulatory. When one functional set dominates a response, it inhibits the development of the other functional set.[55,56] This occurs through the cytokines that are secreted by each cell: IFN-γ and IL-4 are mutually inhibitory. In addition, murine Th1 cell synthesis of IFN-γ is inhibited indirectly by the action of IL-10 on macrophages.[57] Thus, the well-known antithetical relationship between cellular and humoral immune responses in many inflammatory conditions may be explained by the preferential induction and subsequent dominance of either subset.

The factors that determine which type of helper cell will predominate in an immune response are not defined, but they represent an exciting and clinically important area of immunological study. For example, studies of graft infiltrating cells of organ allografts suggest that Th1 cytokine patterns dominate in rejecting grafts, whereas Th2 cytokine patterns are associated with allograft acceptance.[58] If signals could be identified that permit preferential induction of a Th2 pattern of response, appropriate therapies begun during the pretransplant or pretransfusion period might improve graft acceptance rates.

Summary of General Immune Responses

The preceding discussion summarized some newer immunologic concepts that clarify the processes by which the immune system recognizes and responds to foreign antigens. B and T lymphocytes, the cells endowed with receptors to specifically recognize the subtle antigenic variations that distinguish self and nonself antigens, identify these differences through entirely separate mechanisms. B cells "see" foreign epitopes in the antigen's native conformation, whereas T cells "see" the antigen only after it has been processed into discrete peptides and presented on a histocompatibility molecule. T cells not only orchestrate T-cell responses such as DTH and CTL, but also they are essential for most B-cell responses. The types of signals delivered to the T-cell population at the time of antigen recognition may determine both the quantity and the quality of the subsequent responses. If the appropriate signals are not received in a timely fashion, T-cell activation may not occur. Under these circumstances, T cells can develop anergy and not respond to a subsequent specific antigen challenge. Although T cells play a central role in immune responses, none of the responses will occur without an effective system of antigen-presenting cells. The importance of antigen-presenting cells in primary immune responses, especially that of dendritic cells, is increasingly recognized.

The Special Circumstances of Alloimmunization

Self-Reactivity

Most studies that have dissected the immunization process utilized nominal antigens (a term that usually refers to foreign antigens other than MHC molecules). The process of alloimmunization to MHC molecules is less clear, in part because of the special circumstances of generating an immune response to molecules closely related to the host's own antigen-presenting molecules. During the process of T-cell differentiation and maturation within the thymus, the final repertoire of TCR is largely determined by a selection process that is based upon affinity of TCR for self-MHC molecules whose peptide grooves are occupied by various self peptides. T cells with no affinity for self-MHC molecules on thymic epithelial cells receive no signals to clonally expand and will eventually die (no selection). T cells with TCR having any affinity for self MHC receive signals that eventually lead to clonal expansion and differentiation (positive selection). Before expansion proceeds, however, a second, negative, selection process occurs. T cells with high affinity for self MHC presented on thymic medullary macrophage populations receive negative signals that induce cell death. Negative selection is a mechanism to eliminate strong self-reactivity that potentially could result in lethal autoimmune processes. Nevertheless, all remaining positively selected T cells have some binding affinity for self-MHC molecules. The binding affinity of TCR for self-MHC molecules subsequently is augmented when they are expressed in association with appropriate foreign peptides—a process essential for initiating the complex process of antigen-specific T-cell activation.[28(pp 12.3-.5),59-62]

Size of the Alloreactive T-Cell Repertoire

The number of T cells that respond to allogeneic MHC molecules is uniquely large. Relative to nominal antigen reactivity in an immunized individual, precursor frequencies of T-cell alloreactivity in a non-immunized individual is 10-fold greater. This may reflect microheterogeneity of the allogeneic response due to a large array of different peptides that would normally occupy allo-MHC molecules. However, the array of peptides that are presented by a given cell type may not be as large as originally predicted. A recent study of peptides purified and sequenced from a Class II species obtained from a murine cell line found no more than six or seven dominant peptides.[63,64]

It is probable that alloreactivity represents a form of cross-reactivity in which T cells having primary affinity for self-MHC plus peptide x, y, z, etc also display variable affinity for other nonself-MHC molecules. Most investigators now accept the premise that alloreactive T cells are not a unique subset of T cells, but are constellations of cells, each of which is also specific for some other peptide/self-MHC complex (Fig 1-5).[65]

Allorecognition Pathways

Direct Allorecognition

The property of cross-reactive recognition described above implies that some T-cell receptors are able to directly bind to MHC Class I or Class II molecules of allogeneic donor cells without an intervening antigen-processing step. If the allogeneic cell is capable of providing appropriate costimulatory signals (for example, an allogeneic dendritic cell), the T cell would be activated and an immune response could proceed. This mode of recognition, termed "direct allorecogni-

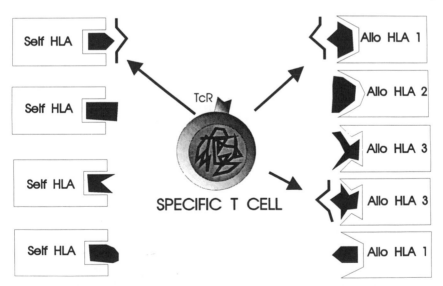

Figure 1-5. A scheme that illustrates the concept of alloreactivity as a form of cross-reactivity. Here, a T-cell receptor that is specific for the conformation formed by self-MHC plus an unknown peptide (upper left self molecule) also cross-reacts with two allogeneic MHC plus peptide complexes with similar conformations. Conformation similarity is denoted by the three black lines drawn over the relevant MHC/peptide complexes.

tion," is unique to MHC alloantigen recognition and is the major pathway responsible for acute cellular rejection of organ allografts.[66] The cellular characteristics of this pathway are direct recognition of MHC Class I/peptide by CD8-positive T cells, or MHC Class II/peptide by CD4-positive T cells, molecules on APCs of "donor" origin, inducing recipient CD8-positive anti-Class I CTL, and CD4-positive anti-Class II CTL or helper cells.

Donor Dendritic Cells in Allorecognition

Passenger leukocytes are known to play a prominent role in acute cellular rejection of allografts.[66] Removal of these mobile cells by "parking" the organ in an immunosuppressed host allows the leukocytes to migrate out of the graft. Survival of the passenger leukocyte-free graft, when transplanted into a secondary recipient of the same strain as the primary immunosuppressed host, is significantly prolonged when compared to a leukocyte-bearing control graft.[65] The principal passenger leukocyte cell type responsible for inducing the acute rejection process appears to be the dendritic cell. When an allograft is transplanted into a recipient, dendritic cells migrate out of the graft and into secondary lymphoid organs of the recipient.[67,68] These cells are thought to migrate into the T-cell zones and initiate a primary immune response via direct allorecognition of foreign MHC Class I or Class II molecules. Thus, donor dendritic cells can bypass the recognition requirement by recipient dendritic cells during early rejection. A similar process may occur when leukocyte-rich platelet products are transfused. Although dendritic cells comprise less than 1% of peripheral blood leukocytes, they have potent APC capacities. Clinical data indicate that platelet preparations effectively depleted of leukocytes reduce the rate of HLA alloimmunization.[69]

Indirect Allorecognition

Alloimmunization to non-HLA alloantigens, such as platelet-specific antigens, is presumed to occur through the standard or indirect allorecognition pathway in which shed platelet alloantigens are taken up, processed and presented to the recipient's T cells by APCs of "recipient" origin. Similarly, shed MHC alloantigens could be taken up by recipient APCs and recognized through the indirect pathway. The role of the indirect alloactivation pathway in presentation of allogeneic MHC antigens is currently a subject of intense interest. Several studies indicate that this pathway is operative in various forms, but its precise in-vivo role in graft rejection or in transfusion-induced alloimmunization needs to be further defined.

A moment's reflection on the presentation of HLA alloantigens via indirect pathways evokes images of a large number of possible presentation pathways. Consider the following permutation in a fully HLA disparate allograft: Recipient dendritic cells could present processed donor Class I or II peptides in the context of recipient Class II molecules; and donor dendritic cells theoretically could present processed self Class I or Class II peptides in the context of either donor Class I or II molecules. (These donor forms of presentation are actually variants of the direct allorecognition pathway.) A number of these presentation pathways have been demonstrated experimentally.[70-74] The current challenge is to determine the role, if any, of indirect alloimmunization in acute cellular rejection and in chronic cellular or humoral rejection.

Minor Histocompatibility Antigens

Genotypically HLA identical sibling transplants are still rejected without immunosuppressive coverage, although the rejection process is less severe. Similarly, acute graft-vs-host-disease (GVHD) regularly occurs in bone marrow transplants performed with genotypically HLA identical sibling donors. Both processes are due to non-HLA or minor histocompatibility transplantation antigens. Definition and physical characterization of minor transplantation antigens have been difficult because few of these antigens induce antibody responses. Recent studies indicate that most of the minor transplantation antigens are endogenously derived peptides that are presented to recipient T cells by donor Class I molecules in organ transplants. (In bone marrow transplants, acute GVHD would be due to recipient Class I molecules presenting peptides to donor T cells.) Two examples of defined minor transplantation antigens are peptides derived from endogenous viruses and the male X-linked H-Y antigen. Not surprisingly, rejection due to this form of minor antigen is mediated by CD8-positive CTL.[75-78] These presentations are variant forms of the direct allorecognition pathway.

Summary and Conclusions

The transfusion or transplantation of allogeneic cells or tissues induces a complex array of immunologic responses geared to elimination of the foreign cells. Major effector responses include CTL with specificity for Class I alloantigens, DTH mediated by Th1 cells and recruited macrophages, and antibodies directed against HLA Class I or Class II molecules. Built into the normal immune response are naturally occurring regulatory circuits that can counter the impact of the pro-inflammatory effector responses. However, these mechanisms usually do not dominate the response unless other modifying influences are imposed. Clinicians traditionally use two strategies to modify the rejection process: 1) immunosuppressive agents that selectively blunt immune effector mechanisms and facilitate the emergence of naturally occurring immune regulatory mechanisms and 2) HLA matching to minimize the number of direct and indirect allorecognition pathways that may be activated.

The immune system is a double-edged sword. Mechanisms that can induce brisk immune effector responses can, under modified conditions, induce negative immune responses or donor-specific acquired tolerance. This premise was recently underscored by Starzl and colleagues[79] who propose a concept, based on the bone marrow chimerism studies of Ildstad and Sachs,[80] that long-term organ allograft acceptance and donor-specific immunosuppression are facilitated by dendritic cells of donor origin that take up residence in recipient lymphoid tissues to create a state of microchimerism and help maintain a state of balanced tolerance.

The challenge in transplantation and the goal of transplantation immunologists are to develop sufficient understanding of the immunologic mechanisms of alloimmunization so that donor-specific immunosuppression can be predictably induced in recipients before or during the early transplant period. It becomes easy to envision a wide breadth of potential new therapeutic interventions based on newer concepts of alloimmunization: monoclonal antibodies against certain adhesion molecules, selective induction of Th2 cells and pharmacologic agents that prevent the migration of donor dendritic cells, to name a few. Many new forms of intervention therapy are under development and will undoubtedly reach clinical trials within 1-2 years.

References

1. Zinkernagel RM, Doherty PC. Restriction of in vitro T cell mediated cytotoxicity in lymphocytic choriomeningitis within a syngeneic or semiallogeneic system. Nature 1974;248:701-2.
2. Bjorkman PJ, Saper MA, Samraoui B, et al. The foreign antigen binding site and T cell recognition regions of class I histocompatibility antigens. Nature 1987;329:512-8.
3. Bretscher PA, Cohn M. A theory of self-nonself discrimination: Paralysis and induction involve the recognition of one and two determinants on an antigen, respectively. Science 1970;163:1042-9.
4. Schwartz RH. A cell culture model for T lymphocyte clonal anergy. Science 1990;248:1349-56.

5. Miller JFAP, Morahan G. Peripheral T cell tolerance. Annu Rev Immunol 1992;10:51-69.
6. Mitchell GF, Miller JFAP. Cell to cell interaction in the immune response. II. The source of hemolysin-forming cells in irradiated mice given bone marrow and thymus or thoracic duct lymphocytes. J Exp Med 1968;128:821-7.
7. Hodgkin PD, Yamashita LC, Coffman RL, Kehry MR. Separation of events mediating B cell proliferation and Ig production by using T cell membranes and lymphokines. J Immunol 1990;145:2025.
8. Noelle RJ, Daum J, Bartlett WC, et al. Cognate interactions between helper T cells and B cells. V. Reconstitution of T helper cell function using purified plasma membranes from activated Th1 and Th2 helper cells and lymphokines. J Immunol 1991;146:1118-24.
9. Noelle RJ, Snow EC. T helper cell-dependent B cell activation. FASEB J 1991;5:2770-6.
10. Lederman S, Yellin MJ, Inghirami G, et al. Molecular interactions mediating T-B lymphocyte collaboration in human lymphoid follicles. Roles of T cell-B cell-activating molecules (Sc8 antigen) and CD40 in contact-dependent help. J Immunol 1992;149:3817-26.
11. Clark EA, Lane PJL. Regulation of human B-cell activation and adhesion. Annu Rev Immunol 1991;9:97-127.
12. Freedman AS, Freeman G, Horowitz JC, et al. B7, a B cell-restricted antigen which identifies preactivated B cells. J Immunol 1987;139:3260-7.
13. Weaver CT, Unanue ER. The costimulatory function of antigen-presenting cells. Immunol Today 1990;11:49-55.
14. Galvin F, Freeman GJ, Razi-Wolf Z, et al. Murine B7 antigen provides a sufficient costimulatory signal for antigen-specific and MHC-restricted T cell activation. J Immunol 1992;149:3802-8.
15. Picker LJ, Butcher EC. Physiological and molecular mechanisms of lymphocyte homing. Annu Rev Immunol 1992;10:561-91.
16. Dustin ML, Springer TA. Role of lymphocyte adhesion receptors in transient interactions and cell locomotion. Annu Rev Immunol 1991;9:27-66.
17. Lassila O, Vainio O, Matzinger P. Can B cells turn on virgin T cells? Nature 1988;334:253-5.
18. Freudenthal PS, Steinman RM. The distinct surface of human dendritic cells, as observed after an improved isolation method. Proc Natl Acad Sci USA 1990;87:7698-702.
19. Steinman RM. The dendritic cell system and its role in immunogenicity. Annu Rev Immunol 1991;19:271-96.
20. Ronchese F, Hausmann B. B lymphocytes in vivo fail to prime naive T cells but can stimulate antigen-experienced T lymphocytes. J Exp Med 1993;177:679-90.

21. Fossum S. The life history of dendritic leukocytes (DL). In: Ivessen OH, ed. Current topics in pathology. Berlin: Springer-Verlag, 1989: 101-24.
22. Romani N, Lenz A, Glassl H, et al. Cultured human Langerhans cells resemble lymphoid dendritic cells in phenotype and function. J Invest Dermatol 1989;93:600-9.
23. Romani N, Inaba K, Witmer-Pack M, et al. A small number of anti-CD3 molecules on dendritic cells stimulate DNA synthesis in mouse T lymphocytes. J Exp Med 1989;169:1153-68.
24. Inaba K, Romani N, Steinman RM. An antigen-independent contact mechanism as an early step in T-cell proliferative responses to dendritic cells. J Exp Med 1989;170:527-42.
25. Liu YJ, Johnson GD, Gordon J, MacLennan ICM. Germinal centers in T-cell-dependent antibody responses. Immunol Today 1992; 13:17-21.
26. Vitetta ES, Berton MT, Burger C, et al. Memory B and T cells. Annu Rev Immunol 1991;9:193-217.
27. Castaño L, Eisenbarth CS. Type I diabetes: A chronic autoimmune disease of human, mouse, and rat. Annu Rev Immunol 1990; 8:647-79.
28. Male D, Champion B, Cooke A, Owen M. Advanced immunology. 2nd ed. London: Gower Medical Publishing, 1991.
29. Bjorkman PJ, Saper MA, Samraoui B, et al. Structure of the human class I histocompatibility antigen, HLA-A2. Nature 1987;329:506-12.
30. Brown JH, Jardetzky T, Saper MA, et al. A hypothetical model of the foreign antigen binding site of class II histocompatibility molecules. Nature 1988;332:845-50.
31. Neefjes JJ, Ploegh HL. Intracellular transport of MHC class II molecules. Immunol Today 1992;13:179-84.
32. Monaco JJ. A molecular model of MHC class-I-restricted antigen processing. Immunol Today 1992;13:173-8.
33. Long EO. Intracellular traffic and antigen processing. Immunol Today 1989;10:232-4.
34. Rudensky AY, Preston-Hurlburt P, Hong SC, et al. Sequence of peptides bound to MHC class II molecules. Nature 1991;353:622-7.
35. Schumacher TNM, de Bruijn MLH, Vernie LN, et al. Peptide selection by MHC class I molecules. Nature 1991;350:703-6.
36. Townsend A, Öhlén C, Bastin J, et al. Association of class I major histocompatibility heavy and light chains induced by viral peptides. Nature 1989;340:443-8.
37. Pfeifer JD, Wick MJ, Roberts RL, et al. Phagocytic processing of bacterial antigens for class I MHC presentation to T cells. Nature 1993;361:359-61.
38. Vitiello A, Potter TA, Sherman LA. The role of β2-microglobulin in peptide binding by class I molecules. Science 1990;250:1423-6.

39. Rock KL, Rothstein LE, Gamble SR, Benacerraf B. Reassociation with β_2-microglobulin is necessary for K^b class I major histocompatibility complex binding of exogenous peptides. Proc Natl Acad Sci USA 1990;87:7517-21.
40. Arnold D, Driscoll J, Androlewicz M, et al. Proteosome subunits encoded in the MHC are not generally required for the processing of peptides bound by MHC class I molecules. Nature 1992;360: 171-4.
41. Momburg F, Ortez-Navarrete V, Neefjes J, et al. Proteosome subunits encoded by the major histocompatibility complex are not essential for antigen presentation. Nature 1992;360:174-6.
42. Tew JG, Kosco MH, Burton GF, Szakol AK. Follicular dendritic cells as accessory cells. Immunol Rev 1990;117:185-211.
43. Gray D, Skarvall H. B cell memory is short-lived in the absence of antigen. Nature 1988;336:70-3.
44. Nunez G, Hockenbury D, McDonnell TJ, et al. Bcl-2 maintains B cell memory. Nature 1991;353:71-3.
45. Noelle RJ, Ledbetter JA, Aruffo A. CD40 and its ligand: An essential ligand-receptor pair for thymus-dependent B-cell activation. Immunol Today 1992;13:431-3.
46. Mosmann TR, Cherwinski H, Bond MW, et al. Two types of murine helper T clone. I. Definition according to profiles of lymphokine activities and secreted proteins. J Immunol 1986; 136:2348-57.
47. Street NE, Mosmann TR. Functional diversity of T lymphocytes due to secretion of different cytokine patterns. FASEB J 1991; 5:171-7.
48. Wierenga EA, Snoek M, de Groot C, et al. Evidence for compartmentalization of functional subsets of CD4+ T lymphocytes in atopic patients. J Immunol 1990;144:4651-6.
49. DelPrete GF, De Carli M, Ricci M, Romagnani S. Helper activity for immunoglobulin synthesis of T helper type 1 (Th1) and Th2 human T cell clones: The help of Th1 clones is limited by their cytolytic capacity. J Exp Med 1991;174:809-13.
50. Salgame P, Abrams JS, Clayberger C, et al. Differing lymphokine profiles of functional subsets of human CD4 and CD8 T cell clones. Science 1991;254:279-82.
51. Romagnani S. Human T_H1 and T_H2 subsets: Doubt no more. Immunol Today 1991;12:256-7.
52. Stevens TL, Bossie A, Sanders VM, et al. Subsets of antigen-specific helper T cells regulate isotype secretion by antigen-specific B cells. Nature 1988;334:255-8.
53. Boom WH, Liano D, Abbas AK. Heterogeneity of helper/inducer T lymphocytes. II. Effects of interleukin-4 and interleukin-2 producing T cell clones on resting B lymphocytes. J Exp Med 1988; 167:1350-63.

54. Greenbaum LA, Horowitz JB, Woods A, et al. Autocrine growth of CD4+ T cells. Differential effects of IL-1 on helper and inflammatory cells. J Immunol 1988;140:1555-60.
55. Pene J, Rousset F, Briere F, et al. IgE production by normal human B cells induced by alloreactive T cell clones is mediated by IL-4 and suppressed by IFN-γ. J Immunol 1988;141:1218-24.
56. Vercelli D, Jobara HH, Lauener RP, Geha RS. IL-4 inhibits the synthesis of IFN-γ and induces the synthesis of IgE in human mixed lymphocyte cultures. J Immunol 1990;144:570-3.
57. Fiorentino DF, Zlotnik A, Vieira P, et al. IL-10 acts on the antigen presenting cell to inhibit cytokine production by Th1 cells. J Immunol 1991;146:3444-51.
58. Lowry RP, Takeuchi T, Cremisi H, Konieczny B. Th2-like effectors may function as antigen-specific suppressor cells in states of transplantation tolerance. Transplant Proc 1993;25:324-6.
59. von Boehmer H. The developmental biology of T lymphocytes. Annu Rev Immunol 1988;6:309-26.
60. Boyd RL, Hugo P. Towards an integrated view of thymopoiesis. Immunol Today 1991;12:71-7.
61. Jorgensen JL, Reay PA, Ehrich EW, Davis M. Molecular components of T-cell recognition. Annu Rev Immunol 1992;10:835-73.
62. Rudensky AY, Rath S, Preston-Hurlburt P, et al. On the complexity of self. Nature 1991;353:660-2.
63. Falk K, Rötzschke O, Stevanović S, et al. Allele-specific motifs revealed by sequencing of self-peptides eluted from MHC molecules. Nature 1991;351:290-6.
64. Gjersten HA, Lundin KEA, Hansen T, Thorsby E. T cells specific for viral antigens presented by HLA-Dw4 recognize DR13 on allogeneic cells: A possible mechanism for induction of rejection. Transplant Proc 1993;25:70-1.
65. Braun MY, McCormack A, Webb G, Batchelor JR. Mediation of acute but not chronic rejection of MHC-incompatible rat kidney grafts by alloreactive CD4 T cells activated by the direct pathway of sensitization. Transplantation 1993;55:177-82.
66. Lechler RI, Batchelor JR. Restoration of immunogenicity to passenger cell-depleted kidney allografts by the addition of donor strain dendritic cells. J Exp Med 1982;155:31-41.
67. Larsen CP, Steinman RM, Witmer-Pack MD, et al. Migration and maturation of Langerhans cells in skin transplants and explants. J Exp Med 1990;172:1483-94.
68. Larsen CP, Morris PJ, Austyn JM. Migration of dendritic leukocytes from cardiac allografts into host spleens: a novel pathway for initiation of rejection. J Exp Med 1990;171:307-14.
69. Kickler TS, Bell W, Drew H, Pall D. Depletion of white cells from platelet concentrates with a new adsorption filter. Transfusion 1989;29:411-4.

70. DeKoster HS, Anderson DE, Termitjelen A. T cells sensitized to synthetic HLA-DR3 peptide gives evidence of continuous presentation of denatured HLA-DR3 by HLA-DP. J Exp Med 1989; 169:1191-6.

71. Chen BP, Madrigal A, Parham P. Cytotoxic T cell recognition of an endogenous class I HLA peptide presented by a class II HLA molecule. J Exp Med 1990;172:779-88.

72. Bradley JA, Mowat AM, Bolton EM. Processed MHC class I alloantigen as the stimulus for CD4+ T-cell dependent antibody-mediated graft rejection. Immunol Today 1992;13:434-8.

73. Fangmann J, Dalchau R, Fabre JW. Rejection of skin allografts by indirect allorecognition of donor class I major histocompatibility complex peptides. J Exp Med 1992;175:1521-9.

74. Benichou G, Takizawa PA, Olson CA, et al. Donor major histocompatibility complex (MHC) peptides are presented by recipient MHC molecules during graft rejection. J Exp Med 1992;175: 305-8.

75. Simpson E. Non-H-2 histocompatibility antigens: Can they be retroviral products? Immunol Today 1987;8:176-8.

76. Rötzschke O, Falk K, Wallny HJ, et al. Characterization of naturally occurring minor histocompatibility peptides including H-4 and H-Y. Science 1990;249:283-7.

77. Wallny HJ, Rammensee HG. Identification of classical minor histocompatibility antigen as cell-derived peptide. Nature 1990; 343:275-8.

78. Roopenian DC. What are minor histocompatibility loci? A new look at an old question. Immunol Today 1992;13:7-10.

79. Starzl TE. Cell migration and chimerism—a unifying concept in transplantation—with particular reference to HLA matching and tolerance induction. Transplant Proc 1993;25:8-12.

80. Ildstad ST, Sachs DH. Reconstitution with syngeneic plus allogeneic or xenogeneic bone marrow leads to acceptance of allografts or xenografts. Nature 1984;307:168-70.

In: Nance ST, ed.
Alloimmunity: 1993 and Beyond
Bethesda, MD: American Association of Blood Banks, 1993

2

The Antibody Response to Antigen

Leslie E. Silberstein, MD

HUMORAL IMMUNITY IS DEFINED by the synthesis of antibody to a specific antigen. The biologic role of antibodies is to neutralize and clear the antigens that induced their formation. The humoral immune response is initiated by activation of individual B cells, followed by differentiation of the B cells into antibody-secreting plasma cells. The resulting antibodies are almost always heterogeneous in structure and specificity, and this diversity can be explained by several factors. First, individual complex antigens can bear multiple antigenic determinants, each of which may activate different B cells. Second, a single antigenic determinant may activate various B cells with slightly different surface immunoglobulin structures (Fig 2-1). Thus, the degree

Complex Antigen   **Simple Antigen**

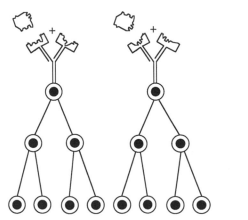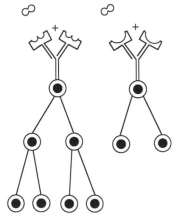

Figure 2-1. Activation of B cells.

Leslie E. Silberstein, MD, Associate Professor, Department of Pathology and Laboratory Medicine, University of Pennsylvania, Philadelphia, Pennsylvania

of antibody diversity will depend on whether the resulting antibodies derive from a single or a few ancestral B cells (eg, monoclonal/oligoclonal antibody population) or from multiple, unrelated B cells (eg, polyclonal antibody population).[1] In general, however, a mixture of antibodies is generated with respect to antibody structure and function. Thus, the characterization of an immune response to alloantigens may address aspects of *clonality, immunoglobulin structure and specificity*; these aspects can be investigated at the protein and/or genetic level.[2]

Phases of the Humoral Immune Response

The sequence of events leading to B-lymphocyte maturation can be categorized into the *antigen-independent* and *antigen-induced* phases. All B cells arise in the bone marrow from CD34 pluripotent progenitor or stem cells that do not synthesize immunoglobulin molecules. The next earliest cell that expresses B-lymphocyte markers is called the *pre-B* cell. This cell expresses cytoplasmic IgM only and no conventional light chains. Consequently, it does not express surface IgM, which requires the association and expression of both heavy and light chains. Therefore, it is believed that pre-B cells do not respond to antigenic stimulation. The next stage of B-cell maturation involves the *immature B cell*, which expresses surface IgM. Once these immature cells leave the bone marrow, they continue to mature and start to express IgD in addition to IgM, and are then

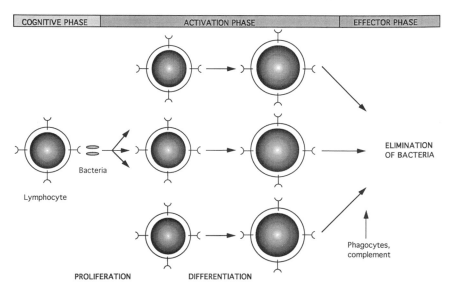

Figure 2-2. Phases of the humoral immune response. (Adapted with permission from Abbas et al.[3])

called *mature B cells* (Fig 2-2). These mature B cells are likely to encounter antigen in the periphery and progress to become *activated B cells*. Activated B cells proliferate and differentiate into *antibody-producing B cells*. During this stage of B-cell differentiation, some B cells will undergo heavy chain isotype switching. Others may not terminally differentiate into plasma cells and, instead, become memory B cells, the stimulation of which leads to secondary antibody responses (see later).

The events leading to antigen-stimulated B-cell differentiation, proliferation and antibody secretion are depicted in Fig 2-3. The initial phase constitutes the cognitive phase, which involves recognition of antigen by B lymphocytes. This phase initiates the proliferation of antigen-specific B-cell clones followed by their differentiation into mature, antibody-secreting plasma cells.

B-Cell Activation/Cognitive Phase

The interaction of B cells with antigen can occur via nonspecific or specific (immunoglobulin) membrane receptors. However, only those B cells whose immunoglobulin receptors have been involved with antigen uptake proliferate and differentiate into antibody-secreting plasma cells. These processes of the humoral immune response depend, to varying degree, on T-cell help. Thus, two major categories of B-cell responses are defined: 1) T-cell independent and 2) T-cell dependent (Fig 2-4). The chemical nature of the inducing antigen (eg, carbohydrate versus protein) plays a major role in determining which of these B-cell responses is initiated.

T-Cell-Independent B-Cell Responses

The definition of these responses comes from animal studies in various mouse strains. There are broadly two types of T-cell-independent antigens.[4] The type 1 T-cell-independent antigen can elicit an immune response in the absence of T-cells or other antigen-presenting cells (discussed later in this chapter). The immune response to type 1 T-cell-independent antigens is largely IgM, IgG2 and IgG3. The type 2 T-cell-independent antigens depends to some degree on T-cell help. From murine studies, it is known that extensive T-cell depletion significantly reduces or abolishes the type 2 immune response to these antigens. However, the addition of small numbers of T cells to the in-vitro cultures restores the responses. Antibodies specific for type 2 T-cell-independent antigens are mostly of the IgM or IgG3 subclass.

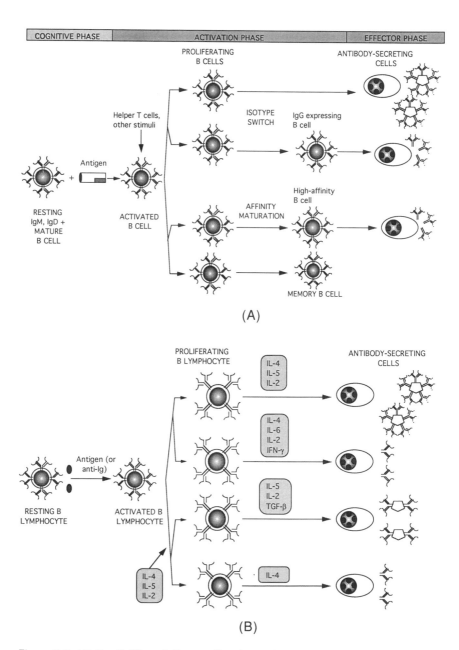

Figure 2-3. (A) B-cell differentiation, proliferation and antibody secretion and (B) role of cytokines. (Adapted with permission from Abbas et al.[3])

The mechanism of B-cell activation by T-cell-independent antigens depends on the type of antigen and its concentration. For example, type 1 antigens (at low concentration only) and type 2 antigens trigger B cells by binding to their antigen-specific immunoglobulin receptors. The interaction of multiple repeating determinants such as those characteristic for many carbohydrate structures cross-links the immunoglobulin receptor, which initiates steps of B-lymphocyte activation (Fig 2-4). At high concentration, however, the type 1 antigens can cross-link *non*immunoglobulin receptors, which are also present on most B cells. However, immunoglobulin receptors may become clustered in this process, leading to B-lymphocyte activation regardless of immunoglobulin specificity. This type of B-cell activation is also referred to as mitogenic stimulation. Since the non-immunoglobulin/mitogen receptors are shared by most B cells, the resulting B-cell response is polyclonal.

T-Cell-Dependent B-Cell Responses

T-cell-dependent antigens are proteins.[4-6] After binding to the immunoglobulin receptor on B lymphocytes, they are endocytosed and processed as in other antigen-presenting cells, such as macrophages. This sequence of events results in the generation of peptide fragments of the antigen, which are subsequently expressed on the surface of the B-cell surface, noncovalently bound to Class II major histocompatibility complex (MHC) molecules.[7] These peptide-MHC Class II complexes can now be recognized by antigen-specific helper T cells. T-cell-independent antigens, on the other hand, are usually carbohydrate in nature and, although they are also taken up by immunoglobulin receptors, these antigens are not processed and subsequently recognized by MHC Class II restricted helper T-cells.

The mechanisms of T-cell and B-cell collaboration in an antigen-specific immune response became better understood from experiments involving hapten-carrier conjugates. Native antigen is first recognized by immunoglobulin receptors via its hapten determinant. Following internalization and processing, the peptide fragments (carrier determinants) are presented in the context of MHC Class II mole-

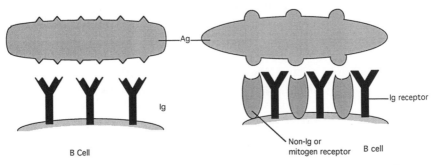

Figure 2-4. T-cell-independent antigens. (Adapted with permission from Abbas et al.[3])

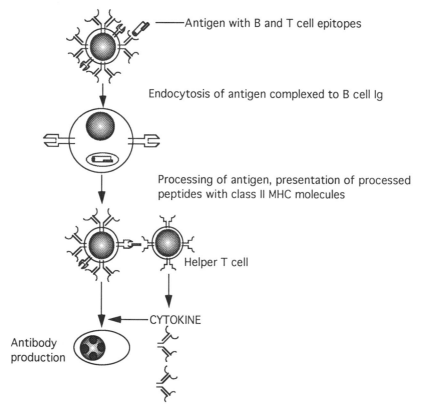

Figure 2-5. T-cell and B-cell collaboration.

cules to specific helper T cells (Fig 2-5). These antigen-specific helper T cells then secrete cytokines that stimulate the proliferation and differentiation of the antigen-specific B cells. The various cytokines play distinct roles during the different stages of B-cell differentiation and proliferation (Fig 2-3). Furthermore, the relative proportion of the different cytokines will influence the nature and magnitude of an immune response because certain cytokines will either synergize or inhibit one another's actions.[3] The type of antigenic stimulus can also influence the degree of T-cell help and thus the production of the various cytokines.

Features of Antibody Responses

Kinetics of Antibody Production

Primary and secondary immune responses refer to the generation of antigen-specific antibody populations during the first and sub-

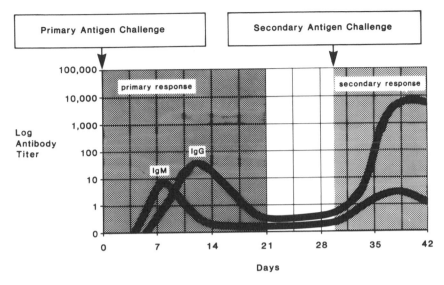

Figure 2-6. Kinetics of antibody production.

sequent exposures of an individual to exogenous antigens. The primary response is characterized by the appearance of antigen-specific IgM antibodies after 5-7 days, followed by IgG antibodies several days later; the titers of both antibodies usually diminish by 28 days.[2] However, upon subsequent challenge with the same antigen, a rapid increase (within 48 hours) in predominantly IgG antibody ensues, which peaks at about 6 days following challenge (Fig 2-6). This sequence of events explains the serologic and clinical manifestations that occur during a delayed hemolytic transfusion reaction.[8]

Clonality of an Antibody Response

The preimmune repertoire (eg, before exposure of an individual to antigen) consists of B cells capable of reacting with a wide variety of antigens. Through the process of clonal selection, however, only those B cells with specificity for a particular antigen are stimulated to proliferate and mature into antibody-secreting plasma cells. Thus, the number of B-cell progenitors that are initially activated and expanded to constitute the immune response to specific antigen determines the subsequent heterogeneity and clonality of the B-cell population specific for that antigen. The clonality of an antibody population ranges from a polyclonal response (eg, following immunization to bacteria or viruses that are capable of simultaneously activating many different B cells) to a monoclonal response (representing the antibody popula-

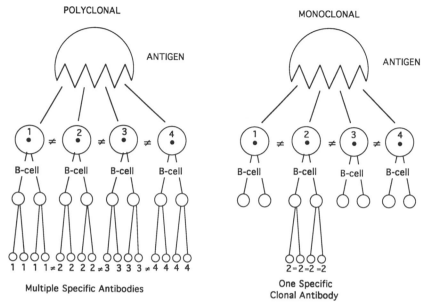

Figure 2-7. Clonality of an immune response.

tion secreted by the progeny of one ancestral B cell) (Fig 2-7). The diversity of immune responses can be examined by analyzing structural and functional aspects at both the protein and genetic level of antibodies and antigen-specific B cells (see below).

Antibody Diversity at the Serologic Level

Specificity (Antigen Binding)

The antibody response, particularly the primary response to a defined antigen, may be quite heterogeneous. In addition to antibodies to the immunizing antigen, one can often detect the emergence of antibodies with unrelated specificities in the serum. Theoretically, even within the antigen-specific antibody response, there exist antibodies to different epitopes of a complex antigen. Studies to define the presence of heterogeneous antibody specificities are not feasible with whole serum because of the low levels of each individual antibody, which makes the isolation of homogeneous antibody populations virtually impossible. To this end, investigators have been establishing B-cell lines in vitro by either Epstein-Barr virus (EBV) transformation or somatic cell hybridization techniques. This approach has been used successfully to generate various B-cell clones specific for red blood cell antigens.

The specificity of the antibodies secreted by these cell lines is determined by conventional red blood cell serology, where the specificity of red cell antibodies is routinely determined by agglutination or solid phase assays. The sensitivity of these agglutination assays can be enhanced by various measures (eg, acidification of serum, proteolytic enzyme treatment of red blood cells). In contrast, solid-phase binding assays do not depend on agglutinability of red cells (with or without the addition of an antiglobulin reagent) and the sensitivity of these solid-phase assays is greatly enhanced by the use of radioactive or enzymatic labels.

Immunoglobulin Structure

Immunoglobulins are divided into five classes on the basis of variations in amino acid composition, carbohydrate content, molecular size and molecular weight. (See Fig 2-8.) These differences are readily identified by serum protein electrophoresis. All immunoglobulins have in common a basic four-chain polypeptide structure consisting of two identical heavy-chain and two identical light-chain subunits covalently linked by disulfide bonds. The heavy chains are divided into five classes (μ, γ, α, δ, ϵ); the light chains may be of two different types (κ or λ). IgG molecules contain two heavy (γ) chains and two light chains (κ or λ); IgM occurs predominantly as pentamers of the

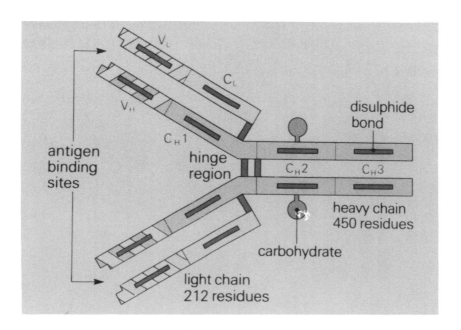

Figure 2-8. Generalized structure of an immunoglobulin molecule.

four-chain structure; and IgA is present as monomers or dimers. Each polypeptide subunit of the four-chain structure is subdivided into various segments. From the amino terminus to the carboxy terminus of the light chains, these segments are, in order, the variable (V), joining (J) and constant (C) regions. The heavy chains also contain a diversity (D) region between the V and J regions. In general, B lymphocytes express only one combination of V(D)J segments throughout their life span. In contrast, C regions of various types (μ, γ, α, etc) can be rearranged to the same V(D)J combination in the ontogeny of a B lymphocyte. The organization of the genes encoding the V, D, J and C regions is discussed later. This molecular rearrangement, termed isotype switching, accounts for the shift in the type of immunoglobulin heavy chain as the immune response to a defined antigen matures.[9,10]

Studies of immunoglobulins were first carried out with serologic reagents that specifically recognized antigenic markers on both heavy- and light-chain polypeptides.[11] The differences between these antigenic markers are illustrated in Fig 2-9.

Isotypes

Genes encoding the various isotypes (ie, IgG, IgM, IgA, IgD, IgE, κ, λ) are all present in the human genome. Antisera specific for isotypic determinants can be prepared by heterologous (across species) immunization (eg, injection of human antibody into a mouse). Isotypes refer to both heavy (class and subclass) and light (type and subtype) chains; they are the result of structural changes confined to the *constant regions* of either heavy or light chains.

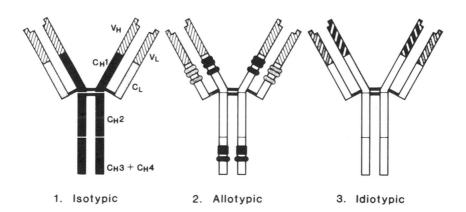

1. Isotypic   2. Allotypic   3. Idiotypic

Figure 2-9. Antigenic markers of immunoglobulin genes.

Allotypes

These distinctions between antibodies are the result of structural polymorphisms in the human genome, and each marker is not present in every individual. This genetic variation can be viewed as resulting from different alleles of a single structural gene locus. Antibodies specific for allotypic variants can be raised by homologous (same species) immunization. Allotypic antibodies are sometimes found in the serum of mothers who have delivered infants with different allotypic markers. Allotypic variants are generally the result of amino acid changes in the antibody constant regions.

Idiotypes

Idiotypic variation is the result of differences in the amino acid structure of the *variable regions* of both heavy and light chains. The target amino acid sequences may lie within the hypervariable or framework regions (Fig 2-9). Anti-idiotypic antibodies may recognize variable region determinants either within or outside the antigen-combining site. Anti-idiotypic antibodies may occur naturally in an individual or they can be induced by either homologous or heterologous immunization. Since anti-idiotypes bind only to a limited subset of B cells, they may be involved in the regulation of a specific immune response. For example, the successful use of intravenous immune globulin (IVIG) therapy in autoimmune thrombocytopenic purpura and for Factor VIII inhibitors has been ascribed to the presence of anti-idiotypic antibodies in the various commercial IVIG preparations.[12]

Characterization of Immunoglobulin Structure

Antibody isotypes and allotypes can be determined with gel electrophoresis followed by immunofixation with the appropriate antisera. Subtle differences in antibody structure, including those resulting in idiotypic differences, can be analyzed by isoelectric focusing. This technique involves gel electrophoresis of serum along a pH gradient until each protein reaches its isoelectric point (ie, the pH at which the antibody protein is electrically neutral).

Genetic Basis for Antibody Diversity

An enormous diversity of antibody specificities already exists prior to antigenic stimulation.[13-16] This preimmune repertoire is defined by the number of B-cell clones ($\sim 10^9$ B lymphocytes) whose specificities are conferred by heavy- and light-chain polypeptide pairing. It is now known that individual heavy- and light-chain polypeptides are not encoded by distinct germ line genes specific for each polypeptide. Instead, B cells dispose of numerous genetic mechanisms for generating a diverse immunoglobulin repertoire from a more limited set of immunoglobulin gene segments in the genome.

Genomic Organization of Immunoglobulin Genes

The organization of immunoglobulin genes is similar in all species.[13,15,17,18] The basic organization of human immunoglobulin genes is illustrated in Fig 2-10. At the 5' end of the heavy- or light-chain locus are located the V(variable) region exons, each about 300 base pairs in length and separated by noncoding DNA segments (introns) of varying length. About 90 base pairs upstream of each V gene is located the leader sequence, which encodes a signal peptide of about 20-30 amino acids. These signal peptides guide the synthesized immunoglobulin peptides into the endoplasmic reticulum, after which they are cleaved off. The number of V gene segments varies for the two light- and one heavy-chain loci; they are organized over large stretches (2000-3000 kilobases). Based on homology, the V gene segments are organized into families. The members of each V gene family share at least 80% nucleotide sequence homology and less than 70% homology with

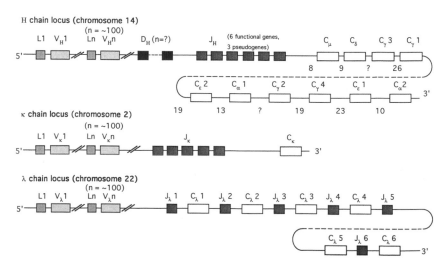

Figure 2-10. Genomic organization of immunoglobulin genes. (Adapted with permission from Abbas et al.[3])

other families. Furthermore, the complexity of each family (eg, the number of *V* gene segment members) differs among the families. In humans, the heavy-chain locus (on chromosome 14) is organized into seven *V* gene families and the κ light-chain locus (chromosome 2) has four families. The λ light-chain locus (chromosome 22) has not yet been fully studied to allow for organization at this time. At varying distances downstream of *V* gene segments are located the joining (J) and diversity (D) region segments and 3′ downstream of these are located the constant region segments.

Immunoglobulin Gene Rearrangement

The recombination (eg, joining) of one *V* gene, one D segment and one J segment to one constant region leads to the transcription and translation of a heavy- or light-chain polypeptide. As shown in Fig 2-11, which illustrates V-D-J joining for the heavy chain, D-J joining is preceded by V-D joining. Thus, the combination of different immunoglobulin gene segments (conferring distinct antigen-binding properties) contributes in part to antibody diversity. Recombination of V_L genes occurs similarly, although *D* gene segments are not involved.

Additional methods of generating antibody heterogeneity involve junctional diversity, which is created by imprecise V-(D)-J joining as illustrated in Figs 2-11 and 2-12 and by N-region insertion. The latter refers to the random addition of nucleotides by the enzyme TdT at the time of V-(D)-J recombination. It is important to note that once a B cell has undergone immunoglobulin rearrangement, its progeny will main-

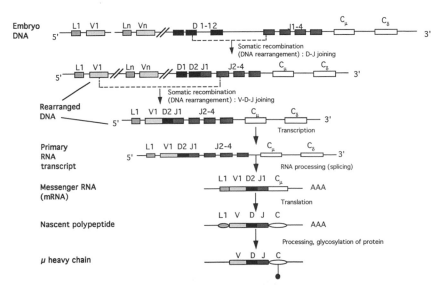

Figure 2-11. Immunoglobulin gene rearrangement. (Adapted with permission from Abbas et al.[3])

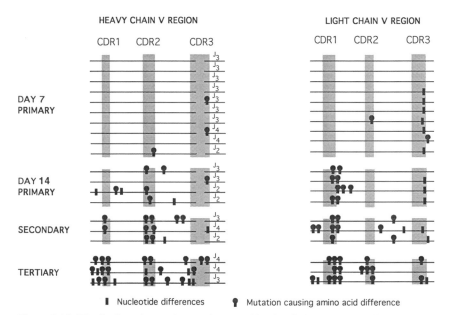

Figure 2-12. Distribution of somatic mutations resulting in affinity maturation. Sequences are derived from hybridomas of immunized mice. (Adapted with permission from Abbas et al.[3])

tain the same rearrangement of heavy- and light-chain genes. Thus, when analyzing clonal populations at the molecular level, one can look for 1) the use of the same *V* gene segments, 2) the same heavy- and light-chain pairing and 3) the same junctional diversity.

Somatic Mutations (Nucleotide Substitutions)

Somatic mutions of immunoglobulin gene segments occur largely following antigenic stimulation.[16] This process often leads to affinity maturation and can also contribute to the generation of a diverse B-cell repertoire. The precise mechanisms of somatic mutations are not known. Studies of primary and secondary immune responses to a defined antigen have revealed the following changes in immunoglobulin gene segments: 1) base pair changes are found overwhelmingly in the *V* gene segments of heavy- and light-chains, 2) the mutations are seen more in IgG than in IgM antibodies and 3) while mutations may occur randomly throughout the *V* gene segment, those that confer amino acid change are found nonrandomly in the hypervariable regions and likely result in affinity maturation (Fig 2-12).

In summary, B cells utilize numerous genetic mechanisms to respond to a large variety of antigens and to fine-tune their antigen-binding properties. As discussed below, the molecular and serologic analyses collectively may provide important biological information on clonality and structure/function correlations.

Heterogeneity of Red Blood Cell Antibodies

It is often difficult to characterize specific antibody populations because of their low serum concentrations. Red-blood-cell-specific antibodies such as cold agglutinins, however, are often present in large quantities in serum as monoclonal immunoglobulins and have been extensively analyzed. Recently, several human monoclonal red blood cell antibodies have been established in vitro, providing a sufficient supply of homogeneous antibody for analysis.

Antigen Binding

As the immune response to a particular antigen matures, the antibodies generated may vary in fine specificity and binding constant. These characteristics are also likely to be applicable to red blood cell antigens, but have been examined only following immunization against Rh antigens. Differences in antigen binding among naturally occurring monoclonal cold agglutinins have also been observed in the serum of an individual. Similarly, serum autoantibodies with "Rh-like" activity may have differential agglutinating reactivity with red cells of varying Rh phenotypes, which also suggests the presence of a heterogeneous serum autoantibody population.[19]

Immunoglobulin Structure

Primary and secondary immune responses to red blood cell antigens have been studied primarily with D-positive red blood cells as the immunogen. The appearance of anti-D following primary immunization varies among individuals.[8] Using standard serologic techniques based on agglutination, it may be 2 weeks to 3 months before anti-D is detected. In addition, the dose of D-positive cells required for primary immunization also varies significantly, from 1 mL up to 200 mL.

Immune responses to the majority of red blood cell alloantigens (Rh, Kidd, Duffy, Kell) are very similar in that the serum contains mostly IgG. Mixtures of IgG, IgM and, rarely, small amounts of IgA may occur. The majority of IgG red blood cell alloantibodies are restricted to the IgG1 and IgG3 subclasses; relatively few belong to IgG2 (anti-A, anti-B and some anti-Rh) and IgG4 (some warm-reactive autoantibodies, anti-Lu^b). Little is known about the relationship of antibody allotypes to red-blood-cell-specific antibodies; the few published studies are limited to Rh antibodies.

In contrast, antibodies of the ABO system are naturally occurring, which suggests immunization against cross-reactive antigens that are widespread on cell types of other organisms such as bacteria. Anti-A and anti-B are predominantly IgM in group B or A individuals, whereas the serum of group O subjects contains significant amounts of anti-A and anti-B that are of the IgG class. The difference in immune response in group O individuals remains unexplained. Other naturally occurring antibodies are found in the Ii, P and MNS systems and are also mostly of the IgM isotype.

Variable Regions

As previously discussed, detailed analyses of antigen-specific immunoglobulin require the isolation of large quantities of homogeneous populations of antibody and/or the generation of relevant in-vitro established cell lines. Therefore, it is not surprising that most progress to date relates to pathologic cold agglutinins, which can be isolated as monoclonal proteins from serum. In addition, it has been feasible to isolate and subsequently immortalize from patients antigen-specific B lymphocytes that secrete the same pathologic antibody as found in the serum. The experimental approach to studying these red cell *auto*antibodies is very relevant to future studies of red cell *allo*antibodies. Therefore, the experimental approach previously used for cold agglutinins is discussed in the remainder of this chapter. In principle, it is first necessary to establish a source of a homogeneous antipopulation. In general, this is accomplished by establishing monoclonal cell lines in vitro. It is then possible to study the V_H and V_L genes at a molecular level and correlate these findings with the structure/function characteristics of the antibodies secreted by the cell lines.

Monoclonal, Pathologic Anti-I/i Cold Agglutinins

Serologic Analyses

Idiotypic variation results from differences in amino acid sequence in both heavy- and light-chain variable regions and anti-idiotypic antibodies can be used to recognize variable region determinants within or outside the antigen-combining site. Through the use of such anti-idiotypic antisera, cross-reactive idiotypes were found among red cell autoantibodies.[20,21] This cross-reactivity appeared to be restricted to red cell autoantibodies with similar specificity. For example, anti-idiotypic antibodies raised against anti-Pr cold agglutinins generally did not cross-react with anti-I cold agglutinins, and vice versa. Subsequent studies by Stevenson et al[22] described a monoclonal anti-idiotypic antibody termed "9G4," which recognized an idiotypic determinant present on the heavy chain of both anti-I and anti-i cold agglutinins as well as on neoplastic B cells secreting cold agglutinins. This suggested that the heavy-chain variable regions of anti-I and anti-i may share some of the same structural elements. Studies from several laboratories[23,24] have found that the 9G4 idiotype is present on all (at least 48/48) pathogenic anti-I/i cold agglutinins studied to date (Table 2-1). As can

Table 2-1. Structural and Idiotypic Diversity of Cold Agglutinin (CA) Assessed With V_H4 Sequence-Dependent Peptide Antibodies and With the 9G4 Reagent[24]

Name	L Chain		H Chain			
	Sequence	V_L	V_H	V_H4-FR1a	V_H4-HV2a	9G4
Anti-I CA						
1. JOH(AJ)	+	$V_\kappa III$	V_H4	NT	NT	NT
2. BAT	−	$V_\kappa III$	V_H4	−	+	+
3. BON	−	$V_\kappa III$	V_H4	+	+	+
4. HIG	−	$V_\kappa III$	V_H4	+	+	+
5. KAU	+	$V_\kappa III$	V_H4	NT	NT	NT
6. LEA	−	$V_\kappa III$	V_H4	+	+	+
7. NAD	−	$V_\kappa III$	V_H4	+	−	+
8. ODO	−	$V_\kappa III$	V_H4	+	+	+
9. PER	−	$V_\kappa III$	V_H4	−	+	+
10. POS	−	$V_\kappa III$	V_H4	NT	NT	NT
11. RIC	−	$V_\kappa III$	V_H4	+	+	+
12. SOC	−	$V_\kappa III$	V_H4	NT	NT	NT
13. TRI	−	$V_\kappa III$	V_H4	NT	NT	NT
14. VOG	+	$V_\kappa III$	V_H4	+	+	+
		$(V_\kappa III)$ 13/14	14/14	7/9	8/9	9/9
Anti-i CA						
1. CAP	+	$V_\kappa I$	V_H4	+	+	+
2. FA	−	$V_\kappa III$	V_H4	+	−	+
3. GRO	−	$V_\kappa III$	V_H4	+	+	+
4. LG	−	$V_\kappa I$	V_H4	+	+	+
5. PER*	−	$V_\kappa \dagger$	V_H4	−	+	−
6. PRO	−	$V_\kappa III$	V_H4	+	−	+
7. RID	−	$V_\kappa III$	V_H4	+	+	+
8. TM	−	$V_\kappa \dagger / V_\lambda$	V_H4	+	+	+
		$(V_\kappa III)$ 4/8	8/8	7/8	6/8	7/8
Non-CA						
1. LES	+	$V_\kappa III$	V_H4	+	−	+
2. SA	−	V_λ	V_H4	−	−	+
3. GRE	−	$V_\kappa III$	V_H4	−	−	+

*Indicates the presence of two different patients with the same initials PER.
†These $_\kappa$ light chains were not reactive with the V_κ family-specific reagents.

be seen in Table 2-1, the 9G4 reagent, although highly associated with anti-i/I cold agglutinins, also binds to rheumatoid factors (eg, LES) encoded by V_H4 genes (non-$V_H4.21$). A structural basis for this idiotypic cross-reactivity could not be fully appreciated at the time because of insufficient data on variable region gene usage that had been derived from amino acid sequences limited to the first framework region.[21] Using primary sequence-dependent polyclonal antibodies to heavy-chain variable region determinants, Silverman et al[25,26] first showed that both the anti-I and anti-i cold agglutinins are derived from a distinct subset of V_H4 family genes.[23]

Molecular V Gene Analyses

More recently, the establishment of EBV-transformed B-cell lines secreting either anti-I or anti-i autoantibodies has allowed for nucleotide sequence analyses of the entire expressed variable region genes to further assess the molecular basis for the autoimmune response.[23,24] Collectively, the work from two laboratories studying four anti-I and two anti-i cold agglutinins indicates that anti-I as well as anti-i cold agglutinins likely derive from the same $V_H4.21$ (or closely related) gene segments (Fig 2-13).[23] Furthermore, protein sequencing of another anti-I cold agglutinin has also indicated $V_H4.21$ usage.[27]

In contrast, the variable region genes used by the anti-I/i light chains do not demonstrate such restriction. While the anti-I cold agglutinin light chains appear to derive from the VkIII gene family, the anti-i cold agglutinins use light chains from a number of different Vk families including VkIII.[23] To determine whether the anti-I/i light chains that use VkIII might exhibit similar idiotypic cross-reactivity as observed for the heavy chains, a panel of eight VkIII light-chain-dependent monoclonal anti-idiotypic antibodies were raised against an anti-I autoantibody expressing V_H4 and VkIII genes.[28] Significant idiotypic heterogeneity was observed among VkIII-expressing cold agglutinin light chains. In addition, the idiotypic heterogeneity could be ascribed to the use of at least three different VkIII gene segments, as well as to somatic diversification of the germ-line-encoded genes.

The expressed variable region genes were also examined for the number and pattern of somatic mutations in order to evaluate the potential role for antigen-mediated selection.[23] It was determined that both the V_H and V_L genes encoding the *anti-i* antibody were identical to germ line sequences, whereas numerous base pair differences were noted in the anti-I response (Fig 2-13). Compared to its most likely germ line precursor, $V_H4.21$, the V_H gene encoding anti-I had only three amino acid differences, two located in framework regions and one in a complementarity determining region (CDR or region of antigen contact). In contrast, the V_L sequence of anti-I had a relatively high number of amino acid substitutions (relative to the total number of

```
            <--------------------------Leader------------------------  <---------------------------Intron-------------------------------
            Met Lys His Leu Trp Phe Phe Leu Leu Leu Val Ala Ala Pro Arg Trp
15B         ATG AAA CAC CTG TGG TTC TTC CTC CTC CTG GTG GCA GCT CCC AGA T   GTGAGTGTCTCA GGAATGCGGATA TGAAGATATGAG ATGCTGCCTCTG ATCCCAGGGCTC ACTGTGGGTT
15A                 --- --- --- --- --- --- --- --- --- --- --- --- --- -
20A                 --- --- --- --- --- --- --- --- --- --- --- --- --- -
20B                 --- --- --- --- --- --- --- --- --- --- --- --- --- -
20C                 --- --- --- --- --- --- --- --- --- --- --- --- --- -

                                            1   2   3   4   5   6   7   8   9  10  11  12  13  14  15  16  17  18  19  20  21  22  23  24  25  26  27
                                Val Leu Ser Gln Val Gln Leu Gln Gln Trp Gly Ala Gly Leu Leu Lys Pro Ser Glu Thr Leu Ser Leu Thr Cys Ala Val Tyr Gly Gly
VH4.21                                      CAG GTG CAG CTA CAG CAG TGG GGC GCA GGA CTG TTG AAG CCT TCG GAG ACC CTG TCC CTC ACC TGC GCT GTC TAT GGT GGG
        ---Intron--->           ----Leader--->
15B     TCTCTGTTCACAG           GG GTC CTG TCC --- --- --- --- --- --- --- --- --- --- --- --- --- --- --- --- --- --- --- --- --- --- --- --- --- ---
15A                             -- --- --- --- --- --- --- --- --- --- --- --- --- --- --- --- --- --- --- --- --- --- --- --- --- --- --- --- --- ---
                                                                                                                    Asn
20A                             -- --- -a- --- --- --- --- --- --- --- --- --- --- --- --- --- --- --- --- --- --- --- -AT --- --c --- --- --- ---
20B                             -- --- -a- --- --- --- --- --- --- --- --- --- --- --- --- --- --- --- --- --- --- --- -AT --- --c --- --- --- ---
20C                             -- --- -a- --- --- --- --- --- --- --- --- --- --- --- --- --- --- --- --- --- --- --- -AT --- --c --- --- --- ---

                  <--------CDR 1-------->                                                                 <------------------CDR 2-----------------
         28  29       30  31  32  33  34  35  36  37  38  39  40  41  42  43  44  45  46  47  48  49  50  51  52  53  54  55  56  57  58  59  60  61  62
        Ser Phe      Ser Gly Tyr Tyr Trp Ser Trp Ile Arg Gln Pro Pro Gly Lys Gly Leu Glu Trp Ile Gly Glu Ile Asn His Ser Gly Ser Thr Asn Tyr Asn Pro Ser
VH4.21  TCC TTC      AGT GGT TAC TAC TGG AGC TGG ATC CGC CAG CCC CCA GGG AAG GGG CTG GAG TGG ATT GGG GAA ATC AAT CAT AGT GGA AGC ACC AAC TAC AAC CCG TCC
15B     --- ---      --- --- --- --- --- --- --- --- --- --- --- --- --- --- --- --- --- --- --- --- --- --- --- --- --- --- --- --- --- --- --- --- ---
15A     --- ---      --- --- --- --- --- --- --- --- --- --- --- --- --- --- --- --- --- --- --- --- --- --- --- --- --- --- --- --- --- --- --- --- ---
                                                         Ala
20A     --- ---      --- --- --- --- --- --- --- --- --- --- G-- --- --a --- --- t-- --- --- --- --- --- --- --- --- --- --- --- --- --- --- --- --- ---
20B     --- ---      --- --- --- --- --- --- --- --- --- --- G-- --- --a --- --- t-- --- --- --- --- --- --- --- --- --- --- --- --- --- --- --- --- ---
20C     --- ---      --- --- --- --- --- --- --- --- --- --- G-- --- --a --- --- t-- --- --- --- --- --- --- --- --- --- --- --- --- --- --- --- --- ---

        -------CDR 2------>
         63  64  65  66  67  68  69  70  71  72  73  74  75  76  77  78  79  80  81  82  83  84  85  86  87  88  89  90  91  92  93  94  95  96  97
        Leu Lys Ser Arg Val Thr Ile Ser Val Asp Thr Ser Lys Asn Gln Phe Ser Leu Lys Leu Ser Ser Val Thr Ala Ala Asp Thr Ala Val Tyr Tyr Cys Ala Arg
VH4.21  CTC AAG AGT CGA GTC ACC ATA TCA GTA GAC ACG TCC AAG AAC CAG TTC TCC CTG AAG CTG AGC TCT GTG ACC GCC GCG GAC ACG GCT GTG TAT TAC TGT GCG AGA
15B     --- --- --- --- --- --- --- --- --- --- --- --- --- --- --- --- --- --- --- --- --- --- --- --- --- --- --- --- --- --- --- --- --- --- ---
15A     --- --- --- --- --- --- --- --- --- --- --- --- --- --- --- --- --- --- --- --- --- --- --- --- --- --- --- --- --- --- --- --- --- --- ---
            Thr
20A     --- -C- --- --- --- --- --t --- --- --- --- --- --- --- --- --- --- --- --a --- --- --- --- --- --- --- --- --- --- --- --- --- --- --- ---
20B     --- -C- --- --- --- --- --t --- --- --- --- --- --- --- --- --- --- --- --a --- --- --- --- --- --- --- --- --- --- --- --- --- --- --- ---
20C     --- -C- --- --- --- --- --t --- --- --- --- --- --- --- --- --- --- --- --a --- --- --- --- --- --- --- --- --- --- --- --- --- --- --- ---
```

Figure 2-13. V gene analysis of anti-i/I cold agglutinins.

silent mutations) when compared to its likely precursor germ line sequence. These amino acid changes resulted from a *nonrandom* distribution of replacement mutations in the CDRs. Taken together, these results provide evidence that positive selection by antigen led to the accumulation of amino acid substitutions in the light chain of the anti-I antibody studied. If this proves to be a universal feature of anti-I cold agglutinins, it may represent a consequence of differential regulation of the immune responses to the related I/i antigens. Perhaps the high expression of i antigen on fetal red cells mediates tolerance to i, either by clonal anergy or deletion of B cells with anti-i specificity. The expression of I antigen occurs much later in development, so immunologic tolerance for I may differ from that for i.

The remarkable restriction in the variable region genes used for the anti-I/i heavy chains and diversification in the associated light-chain variable region gene usage suggest a model for the relative contributions of heavy and light chains to antigen binding. The V_H sequence would be required for the global interaction with the I/i antigen complex, while the V_L sequence would confer the fine specificity that distinguishes between these distinct, yet related, carbohydrate structures. This model for cold agglutinin binding to the I/i antigens is currently being tested through the use of bacterial expression systems that permit the mixing and matching of heavy and light chains from different immunoglobulin molecules. From a practical standpoint, the similarities in idiotypic structure among cold agglutinin heavy-chain variable regions and the ability to generate anti-idiotypic antibodies specific for these structures suggest potential therapeutic applications for these reagents in downregulating the production of autoantibodies or inhibiting the growth of an underlying malignancy.[29-32]

Anti-I/i Cold Agglutinin Isolated From Individuals Without Immune Hemolysis

The issue of what makes an autoantibody clinically significant, ie, pathologic, is another area worthy of investigation. Despite attempts to correlate antibody subclass, complement-fixing ability or antibody titer with the presence or absence of hemolysis, it remains unclear what structural properties distinguish "benign" autoantibodies from hemolytic ones.[33-35] Furthermore, although the spectrum of pathogenic anti-I/i is now known to comprise premalignant clonal B-cell expansions on one end and true malignant lymphomas on the other, it is not known if these clonal disorders have a similar B-cell origin as the natural/benign anti-I autoantibodies. In this regard, this author's laboratory has isolated EBV-transformed anti-I-producing B-cell clones from two normal individuals with a 1:4 cold agglutinin titer in their serum. Sequence analysis of these clones has revealed that if these naturally occurring anti-I cold agglutinins are encoded principally by V_H3 genes (non-$V_H4.21$). This finding indicates that natural anti-i/I specific B cells are not likely to undergo malignant transformation.[36]

Conclusion

Using the approach of EBV transformation followed by cDNA cloning and sequencing of V regions, the diversity of alloantibodies to blood cell elements may be readily accomplished. In this regard, the V regions of several anti-D antibodies have been recently published.[37] As an alternative to the in-vitro establishment of B-cell lines, several nonmammalian expression systems have been developed recently to create human immunoglobulin libraries from which red cell auto- or alloantibodies can be selected. These systems involve the transfection of *Escherichia coli* with human heavy-chain/light-chain constructs that lead to the bacterial secretion of immunoglobulin Fab fragments. Alternatively, heavy-chain/light-chain epitopes that bind antigen can be expressed as part of the viral coat proteins of bacteriophage particles (Winter and Milstein[38] have reviewed these methods). It is anticipated that the generation of appropriate amounts of clonal red cell auto- or alloantibodies using these methods will permit both the analysis of their genetic make-up as well as the identification of the relevant auto/alloantigen molecules.

References

1. Jerne NK. The natural-selection theory of antibody formation. Proc Natl Acad Sci USA 1955;41:849-57.
2. Hood LE, Weissman IL. Immunology. Menlo Park: Benjamin/Cummings, 1978.
3. Abbas AK, Lichtman AH, Pober JS. Cellular and molecular immunology. Philadelphia: WB Saunders, 1991.
4. Finkleman FD, Holmes J, Katona IM, et al. Lymphokine control of in vivo immunoglobulin isotype selection. Annu Rev Immunol 1990;8:303-33.
5. Chestnut RW, Grey HM. Antigen presentation by B cells and its significance in T-B interactions. Adv Immunol 1986;39:51-94.
6. Abbas AK. A reassessment of the mechanisms of antigen-specific T cell-dependent B cell activation. Immunol Today 1988;9:89-94.
7. Lanzavecchia A. Receptor-mediated antigen uptake and its effect on antigen presentation to class II MHC-restricted T lymphocytes. Annu Rev Immunol 1990;8:773-93.
8. Mollison P, Engelfreit C, Contreras M, eds. Blood transfusion in clinical medicine. 9th ed. Oxford: Blackwell, 1993.

9. Davies RD, Padlan EA, Sigal DM, Porter RR. Structural studies of immunoglobulins. Science 1973;180:713-16.
10. Brack B. A complete immunoglobulin gene is created by somatic recombination. Cell 1978;15:1-14.
11. Natvig JB, Kunkel HG. Immunoglobulins: Classes, subclasses, genetic variants and idiotypes. Adv Immunol 1973;16:1-59.
12. Ronda N, Hurez V, Kazatchkine MD. Intravenous immunoglobulin therapy of autoimmune and systemic inflammatory diseases. Vox Sang 1993;64:65-72.
13. Alt FW, Blackwell TK, Yancopoulos GD. Development of the primary antibody repertoire. Science 1987;238:1079-87.
14. French DL, Laskov R. The role of somatic hypermutation in the generation of antibody diversity. Science 1989;244:1152-7.
15. Lai E, Wilson RK, Hood LE. Physical maps of the mouse and human immunoglobulin-like loci. Adv Immunol 1989;46:1-60.
16. Tonegawa S. Somatic generation of antibody diversity. Nature 1983;302:575-81.
17. Berman JE, Alt FW. Human heavy chain variable region gene diversity, organization, and expression. Int Rev Immunol 1990; 5:203-14.
18. Calabi F, Neuberger MS, eds. Molecular genetics of immunoglobulin. Amsterdam: Elsevier Science Publishers, 1987.
19. Petz L, Garratty G. Acquired hemolytic anemia. New York: Churchill Livingstone, 1980.
20. Williams R, Kunkel H, Capra J. Antigenic specificities related to the cold agglutinin activity of gamma M globulins. Science 1968; 161:379-81.
21. Gergely J, Wang AC, Fudenberg HH. Chemical analyses of variable regions of heavy and light chains of cold agglutinins. Vox Sang 1973;24:432-40.
22. Stevenson F, Smith G, North J, et al. Identification of normal B-cell counterparts of neoplastic cells which secrete cold agglutinins of anti-I and anti-i specificity. Br J Haematol 1989;72:9-15.
23. Silberstein LE, Jefferies LC, Goldman J, et al. Variable region gene analysis of pathologic human autoantibodies to the related i and I red blood cell antigens. Blood 1991;73:272-86.
24. Pascual V, Vistor K, Leisz D. Nucleotide sequence analysis of the V regions of two IgM cold agglutinins: Evidence that the V_H4-21 gene segment is responsible for the major cross-reactive idiotype. J Immunol 1991;146:4385-91.
25. Silverman GJ, Goldfien RD, Chen P, et al. Idiotypic and subgroup analysis of human monoclonal rheumatoid factors. J Clin Invest 1988;82:469-75.
26. Silverman G, Goni F, Fernandez J. Distinct patterns of heavy chain variable region subgroup use by human monoclonal autoantibodies of different specificity. J Exp Med 1988;168:2361-6.

27. Leoni J, Ghiso J, Goni F, Froangione B. The primary structure of the Fab fragment of protein KAU, a monoclonal immunoglobulin M cold agglutinin. J Biol Chem 1991;266:2836-42.
28. Jefferies L, Silverman G, Carchidi CM, Silberstein L. Idiotypic heterogeneity of $V_k$iii-restricted cold agglutinin light chains. Clin Immunol Immunopathol 1992;65(2):119-28.
29. Kelsoe GM, Reth M, Rajewsky K. Control of idiotype expression by monoclonal anti-idiotype antibodies. Immunol Rev 1980;52: 74-88.
30. Campbell MJ, Carroll E, Kon S. Idiotype vaccination against murine B cell lymphoma. Humoral and cellular responses by tumor-derived immunoglobulin M and its molecular subunits. J Immunol Methods 1987;139:2825-33.
31. Miller RA, Maloney D, Warnke R. Treatment of B-cell lymphoma with monoclonal anti-idiotypic antibodies. N Engl J Med 1982; 306:517-22.
32. Meeker TC, Lowder J, Maloney D. A clinical trial of anti-idiotypic therapy for B cell malignancy. Blood 1965;65:1349-63.
33. Garratty G. The significance of IgG on the red cell surface. Transfus Med Rev 1987;1:47-57.
34. Rosse W, Adams J. The variability of hemolysis in the cold agglutinin syndrome. Blood 1980;56:409-16.
35. Schreiber A, Herskovitz B, Goldwein M. Low-titer cold hemagglutinin disease mechanism of hemolysis and response to corticosteroids. N Engl J Med 1977;296:1490-4.
36. Jefferies LC, Carchidi CM, Silberstein LE. Naturally occuring anti-i/I cold agglutinins may be encoded by different V_H3 genes as well as the $V_H4.21$ gene segment. J Clin Invest (in press).
37. Hughes-Jones NC, Bye JM, Beale D, Coadwell J. Nucleotide sequence and three-dimensional modelling of the V_H and V_L domains of two human monoclonal antibodies specific for the D antigen of the human Rh-blood group system. J Biol Chem 1990; 268:135-40.
38. Winter G, Milstein C. Man-made antibodies. Nature 1991;349: 293-9.

In: Nance, ST, ed.
Alloimmunity: 1993 and Beyond
Bethesda, MD: American Association of Blood Banks, 1993

3

Granulocyte Alloantigen Systems and Their Clinical Significance

Jeffrey McCullough, MD; Mary E. Clay, MS, MT(ASCP);
and David F. Stroncek, MD

MORE THAN 70 YEARS AGO, Doan reported that the sera of some individuals caused agglutination of the leukocytes of others.[1] It was almost 40 years later that Lalezari, studying neutropenic newborns, described granulocyte-specific antibodies and antigens.[2,3] Subsequently, it has been shown that these antigens and antibodies have important medical effects.[4] This chapter will update the information about the clinical relevance of these antigens and antibodies.

Granulocyte Antigen Systems

Some of the major advances in understanding granulocyte antigens have come through the application of newer techniques of molecular biology and biochemistry. For example, the structure and composition of several of these antigens and their relationship to other molecules of importance on the granulocyte surface are now known.

Jeffrey McCullough, MD, Professor, Department of Laboratory Medicine and Pathology and Director, Division of Laboratory Medicine and Section of Transfusion Medicine, University of Minnesota Hospital, Minneapolis and Scientific Director, American Red Cross Blood Services, St. Paul Region, St. Paul; Mary E. Clay, MS, MT(ASCP), Administrative Scientist, Blood Bank, Department of Laboratory Medicine and Pathology, University of Minnesota Hospital, Minneapolis, and Director, Research and Development Department, American Red Cross Blood Services, St. Paul Region, St. Paul; and David F. Stroncek, MD, Assistant Professor, Department of Laboratory Medicine and Pathology and Medical Director, Blood Bank, University of Minnesota Hospital, Minneapolis and Associate Medical Director, American Red Cross Blood Services, St. Paul Region, St. Paul, Minnesota

Granulocyte Alloantigens

The first granulocyte-specific antigen identified has become known as NA1. This antigen was found when it was shown that the serum of a woman who delivered a neutropenic infant agglutinated the leukocytes of her husband and the infant, but not her own cells.[2] As described by Lalezari, this clinical situation is the neutrophil (granulocyte) equivalent of the red cell hemolytic disease of the newborn. Subsequently, antigens have been identified to additional systems and those found to be unique to granulocytes have been given a standard nomenclature: N standing for neutrophil; then the letters, A, B, C, etc, to designate each different antigen system or apparent genetic locus; then a number to indicate each different allele in that system or at that genetic locus (Table 3-1). Antigens that are shared with other cells or

Table 3-1. Granulocyte Antigens Identified by Human Alloantibodies

Locus	Antigen	Antigen Frequency*	Gene Frequency*
Granulocyte-specific antigens:			
NA	NA1	46	0.37
	NA2	88	0.63
	NA null		
NB	NB1	97	0.83
	NB2	32	0.17
NC	NC1	91	0.72
ND	ND1	nd	nd
NE	NE1	nd	nd
Granulocyte antigens shared with other tissues:			
5	5a	33	0.18
	5b	97	0.82
9	9a	58	0.35
Mart	MART	99	0.91
Unclassified granulocyte antigens:			
CN1			
KEN			
LAN			
LEA			
SL			

*American population
nd = not determined

that remain unclassified have not been given these designations since this nomenclature system is reserved for antigens that are unique to neutrophils.

Granulocyte antigens include those that are unique to granulocytes (and not found on other cells), those that are shared with other cells and a few individual unclassified antigens identified by particular sera whose distribution is not known. All of these antigens were found using traditional blood group serologic techniques such as agglutination, immunofluorescence or cytotoxicity. Monoclonal antibodies are now available that also detect some of these. There are five antigen systems that are unique to granulocytes, three that are shared with other tissues and four unclassified antigens.

The NA system has been studied most extensively. There is a biallelic relationship between NA1 and NA2 with rare individuals who appear to be NA null. It is thought that there may be a third (silent) allele at this locus.[5,6] At least some of these apparently NA null individuals lack the FcRIII molecule, which contains the NA antigens. In the NB system, it is not clear whether the antigen NB2 is in fact the allele of NB1. Studies of gene frequencies and variability in reactivity of sera do not provide clear-cut answers.[7] Alleles for NC, ND and NE have not been reported.

Biochemistry of Granulocyte-Specific Antigens

The NA1 and NA2 antigens are part of the FcRIII molecule, which is a glycoprotein with a molecular weight ranging from 50 to 80 kDa, depending on the NA status of the individual.[8-10] Most of the difference in molecular weight between NA1 and NA2 individuals is due to differences in the amount of carbohydrate on each molecule. The FcRIII molecule has only an extracellular domain and belongs to the group of glycoproteins attached to the membrane by a lipid glycosylphosphatidylinositol (GPI) anchor. This type of linkage allows the molecule to be highly mobile and the FcRIII molecule containing NA antigens is released into the plasma following stimulation of the cells with chemotactic agents.[11] The NB1 antigen is a 58 to 64-kDa plasma membrane glycoprotein that, like the FcRIII (NA) molecule, is linked to the membrane by a GPI anchor.[12-14]

Molecular Biology of Granulocyte-Specific Antigens

The gene that determines the NA1 and NA2 FcRIII molecule has been cloned.[15,16] Both NA1 and NA2 are composed of 233 amino acids but their sequences differ by six amino acids. It has been hypothesized that these amino acid changes mask the NA1 epitope in NA2 individuals. FcRIII is also found on natural killer (NK) cells, but NK cells do not contain the NA or NB antigens.[15] The NK cell FcRIII gene encodes an additional 21 C-terminal amino acids that contribute both to the processing of this protein, from a GPI-linked molecule on granulocytes, to a longer transmembrane-anchored protein on NK cells and to its different function on NK cells vs granulocytes.

Granulocyte Cytoplasmic Antigens

The antigens listed in Table 3-1 are found on the surface of the cell. For years, it has been known that there are also granulocyte-specific antigens in the cell cytoplasm.[17,18] About 10 years ago, a relationship was established between these granulocytoplasmic antigens and the autoimmune disease Wegener's granulomatosis.[19,20] The antibodies to these cytoplasmic antigens are now called antineutrophil cytoplasmic antibodies (ANCA), and they have been shown to be involved in several autoimmune diseases including: systemic necrotizing vasculitis, polyarteritis nodosa, renal disease (idiopathic crescentric glomerulonephritis), Churge-Strauss syndrome and some other poorly characterized diseases.[7,21] Thus, ANCA are valuable serologic markers for vascular inflammatory diseases. The two most important antigens recognized by ANCA are proteinase 3 and myeloperoxidase. These molecules are present in the primary granules and, after granulocyte activation, they are translocated to the cell surface where they can be detected. Other molecules recognized by ANCA include: elastase, lactoferrin, cathepsin G, peroxidase and CAP 57 (an antimicrobial protein). The significance of ANCA reactive with these molecules is not known.

ANCA may have a cytoplasmic (C-ANCA) or perinuclear (P-ANCA) staining pattern. The C-ANCA generally reacts with proteinase 3 and are found more commonly in patients with Wegener's granulomatosis, while the P-ANCA react generally with myeloperoxidase and are found more commonly in patients with renal disease.[7]

Granulocyte Antigens Defined by Monoclonal Antibodies

Numerous monoclonal antibodies have been produced that identify human granulocyte antigens. Some of these monoclonal antibodies detect antigens unique to granulocytes and other reagents define antigens that are common to granulocytes, other cells and tissue. Although many of these determinants appear to serve operationally as differentiation markers, some represent epitopes on functionally significant membrane proteins. Examples are: CR3, C3bi, Fc receptor for IgG and the lymphocyte function-associated (LFA) antigens, which function as leukocyte adhesion molecules. The antigens listed in Tables 3-2 and 3-3 represent granulocyte antigens of current interest and investigation that have been identified with monoclonal antibodies.[20] The clusters of differentiation (CD) as defined by the Fourth International Workshop and Conference on Human Leukocyte Differentiation Antigens[23] are shown along with some basic information about their functional and biochemical characteristics. Only five of the many granulocyte monoclonal antibodies thus far reported have shown absolute or preferential specificity for the polyclonal serologically defined granulocyte antigens, and these antibodies appear to be directed against the NA1, NA2 and NB1 antigens.[7] CLB-gran 11, with specificity for the NA1 antigen, was originally discovered during an analysis of monoclonal antibodies produced against the granulocyte FcRIII.[8] Subsequently, this same group described another monoclonal antibody (GRMI)[24] that reacts preferentially but not specifically with NA2-positive granulocytes.[22] Additional monoclonal antibodies that react specifically (MG38)[25] or preferentially (B73.1)[22] with NA1-positive granulocytes have been reported. Only one monoclonal antibody directed against the NB1 antigen has been produced thus far,[26] but it has been a valuable reagent for NB1 biochemical and cellular distribution studies.[13]

Heterogeneous Expression of Some Granulocyte Antigens

Some granulocyte antigens are detected on some but not all granulocytes, thus creating subpopulations of cells. The antibodies that show a heterogeneous reaction and, thus, define subpopulations of granulocytes include several monoclonal antibodies and NB1 allosera.[7] When techniques such as elutriation have been used to separate the granulocyte subpopulations, differences in chemotaxis, production of toxic oxygen products, depolarization and rosette formation are found.[7] At least one of these antigens, 31D8, changes as the cell matures and, thus, may be a differentiation marker. The implication of these heterogeneous antigens is not completely understood, but continues to be a source of interesting study of the physiology and structure of granulocytes.

Molecules of the Granulocyte Membrane

The molecules important in the granulocyte membrane include: blood group antigens (such as HLA), chemotactic receptors, phagocytic receptors, complement receptors, cell adhesion molecules and mole-

Table 3-2. Representative Granulocyte Antigens Identified With Murine Monoclonal Antibodies—I

Ab/Ag Cluster Designation	Recognized Membrane Antigen	Antigen MW (kDa)	Ligand
CD10	CALLA	gp100	—
CD11a	α chain of LFA-1	gp180	ICAM-1
			ICAM-2
CD11b	α chain of CR3 (Mac-1, Mo1)	gp165	C3bi
			Fibrinogen
			Coagulation factor x
			Endotoxin
CD11c	α chain of CR4 (gp 150/95)	gp150	C3bi
CD15	X-hapten (3-FAL, Lewis X)	gp 50, 68, 110, 180	—
CD16	FcRIII	gp 50–65	IgG (complexed)
CD18	β chain of LFA-1, CR3, CR4	gp 95	(same as CD11 a,b,c ligands)
CD29	β chain of VLA-6 (a6 β1)	gp 120–150	Laminin
CD31	Platelet endothelial cell adhesion molecule-1 (PECAM-1)	gp 130–140	—
CDw32	FcRII	gp 40	IgG (aggregated)
CD44	H-CAM (Hermes antigen)	gp 80–95	Endothelial cell mucosal addressin
			Type I collagen
			Type VI collagen
CD45	LCA (T200)	gp 180, 190, 205, 220	—
CD49f	A chain of VLA-6 (a6 β1)	gp 120	Laminin
CD55	DAF	gp 70	C3b, C4b
CD64	FcRI	gp 75	IgG (monomeric)

CD groups have not
been assigned for
the following
monoclonal
antibodies:

CLB-gran 11, MG38	NA1	gp 45-60	—
B73.1*			
GRM1*	NA2	gp 60-75	—
1B5	NB1	gp 58-64	—
gp-100^MEL-14	LEC-CAM adhesion protein	gp 100	Endothelial cell carbohydrate

*These molecules are neither granulocyte-specific nor absolutely NA allotype-specific.[22]
Ab/Ag = antibody/antigen; CALLA = common acute lymphoblastic leukemia antigen; C3b = complement protein 3b; C3bi = proteolytic fragment of complement protein C3; C4b = complement protein 4b; CR3 = complement (C3) receptor 3; CR4 = complement (C3) receptor 4; DAF = decay accelerating factor; 3-FAL = 3-fucosyl-N-acetyllactosamine; FcRI = Fc receptor I for IgG; FcRII = Fc receptor II for IgG; FcRIII = Fc receptor III for IgG; H-CAM = homing-cell adhesion molecule also known as the Hermes antigen; ICAM-1 = intercellular adhesion molecule-1; ICAM-2 = intercellular adhesion molecule-2; LCA = leukocyte common antigen; LEC-CAM = lectin-epidermal growth factor (EGF)-complement-cell adhesion molecule; LFA-1 = leukocyte function antigen-1; Lewis X = Lewis X antigen; Mac-1/Mo1 = initial monoclonal antibodies that identified the CD11b molecule; this antigen is often referred to as Mac-1 or Mo1; PECAM-1 = platelet endothelial cell adhesion molecule-1; VLA-6 = very late antigen-6.

(Reprinted with permission from Clay ME, Stroncek DF.[7])

Table 3-3. Representative Granulocyte Antigens Identified With Murine Monoclonal Antibodies—II

Ab/Ag Cluster Designation	Antigen Function
CD10	Neutral endopeptidase (enkephalinase)
CD11a	Integrin receptor
	Leukocyte-leukocyte adhesion
	Leukocyte-endothelial cell adhesion
CD11b	Integrin receptor
	Cell-cell adhesion (PMN-endothelial cell adhesion)
	Phagocytosis
	Complement binding
CD11c	Integrin receptor
	Complement binding
CD15	Possible ligand for selectins
CD16	Low affinity Fc receptor for complexed IgG (ie, immune complexes)
	Main receptor for ADCC
	Cross linked antibodies can activate cytotoxicity, cytokine production and receptor expression
CD18	(same as CD11 a,b,c functions)
CD29	Laminin receptor
CD31	Cell-cell adhesion
	Immunoglobulin gene superfamily adhesion molecule
CDw32	Low affinity Fc receptor for aggregated IgG
	Cell activation molecule
CD44	Cell-cell adhesion
	Homing receptor
CD45	Signal transduction molecule
	Tyrosine phosphatase
CD49f	Laminin receptor
CD55	Complement regulation
CD64	High affinity Fc receptor for IgG
	Transduces activation signals

CD groups have not been assigned for the following monoclonal antibodies:

CLB-gran 11, MG38, B73.1*	Unknown; located on neutrophil FcRIII (CD16)
GRM1*	Unknown; located on neutrophil FcRIII (CD16)
1B5	Unknown
gp-100[MEL-14]	Initial adhesion of granulocytes to endothelial cells adjacent to inflammation

*These molecules are neither granulocyte-specific nor absolutely NA allotype-specific.[22]
Ab/Ag = antibody/antigen; ADCC = antibody-dependent cell-mediated cytotoxicity; FcRIII = Fc receptor III for IgG; PMN = polymorphonuclear leukocytes.

(Reprinted with permission from Clay ME, Stroncek DF.[7])

cules important for the structural integrity of the cell. It appears that some of the granulocyte-specific antigens are part of either phagocytic receptors, chemotactic receptors or cell adhesion molecules and, thus, a brief description of these molecules and their relationship to granulocyte-specific antigens will be provided here.

Complement Receptors

The best-characterized granulocyte complement receptors are CR1, CR3 and C5a. Both CR1 and CR3 are responsible for granulocyte phagocytic and adhesive properties. The C5a receptor mediates chemotaxis to complement component C5a. CR1 binds cleavage fragments of C4 and C3 and is made up of 30 short consensus repeats.[27] CR3 is a member of the integrin family and binds C3bi.[28]

Chemotactic Receptors

One of the special functions of granulocytes is the ability to respond to and move toward chemical stimuli. This process of directed locomotion, chemotaxis, is a response to certain bacterial products, complement components, products of damaged tissues and other factors. The surface of the granulocyte contains molecules that are receptors for chemotactic agents, including f-met-leu-phe (FMLP), C5a, interleukin 8 (IL-8) and platelet-activating factor (PAF).[29-31]

The structure of these chemotactic receptors is related. They belong to the G-protein-coupled receptor superfamily and initiate signal transduction via guanine nucleotide-binding regulator proteins (G-proteins). The FMLP receptor has been best characterized. It crosses the plasma membranes seven times, forming three extracellular and three intracellular loops. The C5a and IL-8 receptor genes have been cloned and sequenced and both are similar to the FMLP receptor.[30,31] The amino acid sequence of the C5a receptor expresses 35% homology with the FMLP receptor.[30]

Phagocytic Receptors

Another special function of granulocytes is the ability to attach themselves to foreign material and to ingest and destroy it. The attachment and ingestion, or phagocytosis, involve specific surface molecules that serve as receptors for the foreign material and cause the cell to begin the active process of ingestion. These phagocytic receptors include the Fc receptors FcRII and FcRIII, and complement receptors CR1 and CR3.

Cell Adhesion Molecules

Integrins

Integrins play a key role in development, the immune response, platelet aggregation, tissue repair and possibly hematopoiesis. Integrins are a group of cell membrane glycoproteins with an alpha and a beta subunit. Eleven different alpha subunits and six different beta subunits have been described.[32] The alpha chain contains a calcium-binding region and the beta chain contains four cysteine-rich repeats. The extracellular domains of the alpha and beta subunits contain the ligand-binding region. The cytoplasmic portion of the beta subunits contains regions capable of binding to cytoskeletal actin.[7] There are three different types of granulocyte integrin molecules: leukocyte function antigen-1 (LFA-1), CR3 and p150/95. All have the same β chain, B2, but different α chains and are sometimes referred to as the B2 integrins. Lack of these integrins is an autosomal inherited disorder called leukocyte adhesion deficiency. Affected individuals have recurrent infections, impaired wound healing, diminished pus formation and granulocytosis.

In lymphocytes, LFA-1 mediates cell adhesion and a wide variety of events, including interactions with endothelial cells and cytotoxic T-cell-mediated cell lysis.[28] In granulocytes, LFA-1 is especially important in the adhesion of granulocytes to endothelial cells by interaction with the endothelial cell adhesion molecules ICAM-1 and ICAM-2. Expression of ICAM-1 is increased on endothelial cells by stimulation with certain mediators of inflammation. A congenital lack of the LFA-1 molecule results in severe leukocyte adhesion deficiency and the patients have recurrent serious infections.[33,34]

The granulocyte integrin molecule CR3 is the receptor for the complement component C3bi.[35,36] This receptor binds not only complement but also fibrinogen, coagulation Factor X and endotoxin, and is activated by cardiopulmonary bypass.[37] The CR3 receptor, therefore, is involved in phagocytosis, complement binding and cell adhesion.

The third granulocyte integrin, p150/95, also binds C3bi, but its function is not understood. Both CR3 and p150/95 have increased expression following stimulation with the chemotactic agent FMLP.

Selectins

In order for neutrophils to move to a site of inflammation, they must first adhere to the vascular endothelium, then move through the endothelium and migrate to the site of inflammation. The initial contact between the granulocyte and the endothelium is mediated by a family of molecules called selectins. The selectin molecules are present on the endothelial cells and the ligands for these selectins are on the surface of granulocytes. The carbohydrate ligand on the surface of granulocytes that reacts with both of these selectins includes the Lewis X antigen,[38] although the ligands themselves are slightly different.[39] All selectins have a common structure consisting of an N-terminus lectin-binding domain, an epidermal growth factor-like domain and a varying number of short repeat motifs that are similar to those in complement regulatory proteins.[7] There are three types of selectins: E-selectin, P-selectin and L-selectin. The E-selectins are located on endothelial cells, the P-selectins on platelets and L-selectins on lymphocytes.[40] The L-selectin MEL-14 is a peripheral lymph node-endothelial homing receptor.[41] The L-selectin leukocyte adhesion molecule-1 (LAM-1) controls the binding of lymphocytes to endothelial venules of peripheral lymph nodes and is expressed on granulocytes. Its expression is first increased but later decreased when granulocytes are stimulated with PMA, chemotactic factors, leukotriene, GM-CSF and TNF.[42-44] Two other selectins involved in granulocyte endothelial binding are located on endothelial cells and/or platelets [ie, E-selectin (ELAM-1) and P-selectin (GMP-140)], but they recognize carbohydrate ligands on the surface of granulocytes.

Other cell adhesion molecules located on granulocytes include CD44 and PECAM-1. Their role in granulocyte function or structural integrity is not known and no granulocyte antigens are known to be associated with these molecules.

Relationship of Granulocyte Antigens to Other Granulocyte Membrane Molecules

As with other blood cells, granulocyte antigens are sometimes located on parts of molecules that are important for structural integrity or function. For instance, the receptor for the malaria parasite and the Duffy blood group antigen are part of the same molecule and the molecule containing the Rh antigen is an important structural component of the red blood cell membrane because Rh_{null} individuals have abnormally shaped cells and a hemolytic anemia.

In granulocytes, the antigens NA1 and NA2 are located on FcRIII,[8,9] a key molecule in phagocytosis. Decreased expression of granulocyte-specific antigens has been reported in patients with chronic myelogenous leukemia and paroxysmal nocturnal hemoglobinuria (PNH) and in preterm neonates. The FcRIII molecule is deficient in patients with PNH and, thus, they present with an "NA_{null}" phenotype.[9] Inherited lack of the FcRIII molecule (and, thus, the NA antigens) has also been reported.[27] Except for the one person with systemic lupus erythematosus (SLE),[45] these individuals were healthy and had no evidence of increased susceptibility to infections. In several of these people, the FcRIII gene was defective or absent.[45]

Polymorphisms of the integrins LFA-1 and CR3 have also been described.[7] At least two granulocyte antigens are located on these important molecules. The alloantigen Ond is located on LFA-1 and the alloantigen Mart is located on CR3.[46] The structural or biochemical differences in the LFA-1 and CR3 molecules that account for these polymorphisms are not known. Also, it is not clear whether this polymorphic or structural portion of the integrin molecule is important to granulocyte function. Thus, it cannot yet be concluded whether the polymorphism for these epitopes (antigenic determinants) is important in granulocyte function.

Although there is no evidence that NB1 is part of the molecule that is the receptor for the chemotactic agent FMLP, NB1-negative individuals have a reduced FMLP chemotactic response compared to NB1-positive individuals and NB1-negative cells respond to FMLP to a lesser degree than NB1-positive cells.[47] No other granulocyte-specific antigens are known to be associated with chemotactic receptors or alterations in chemotaxis. Thus, continued study of granulocyte-specific antigens can be expected to provide information about structure and function of the cell itself.

Granulocyte Antibodies

Granulocyte antibodies can be categorized in several ways, many of which overlap; however, they are convenient ways to consider these antibodies. The various methods for detecting granulocyte antibodies were reviewed extensively in 1985[48] and published in more detail,[49] but have not changed appreciably since. Those reviews remain timely.

Serologic Behavior

Because of the number of different kinds of molecules on the surface of granulocytes, several different techniques have been used to detect antibodies against granulocyte surface molecules (Table 3-4). In addition, some of these techniques have a number of different variations that alter the sensitivity of the assay and, thus, provide different results when populations are screened or when a particular person is tested. This has sometimes made it difficult to compare the results of different studies. In addition, there are some methodologic requirements for working with granulocytes that make granulocyte antibody testing difficult, time-consuming and costly. For instance, most of the assays require the use of fresh granulocytes; granulocytes have a natural tendency to ingest foreign material with which they come in contact.

Immunochemistry

Most granulocyte antibodies are IgG, but this may be influenced by the fact that agglutination has been the method most commonly used for their detection and agglutination detects IgG antibodies. In other words, leukoagglutinating antibodies are usually IgG. Granulocytoxins are usually IgM, but occasionally may be IgG.[81] It is difficult to determine whether there is a relationship between the immunochemical make-up and the clinical effect of granulocyte antibodies. Both IgG

Table 3-4. Granulocyte Antibody Detection Methods

General Phenomenon	Specific Technique
Agglutination of granulocytes	Agglutination Macroscopic[2,50] Microscopic[51,52] Microcapillary[53-55]
Antibody coating of granulocytes	Cytotoxicity Complement-mediated Dye (Eosin) exclusion[56-59] Fluorochromasia[60,61]
	Cell-mediated ADLG (antibody-dependent lymphocyte-mediated granulocyte) cytotoxicity[62-64]
	Immunofluorescence Macroscopic[65-67] Microscopic[68,69] Flow cytometry[70]
	ABC (avidin-biotin complex) immunoassay[71] ELISA (enzyme-linked immunosorbent assay)[72] Radioimmunoassay[73-75] Staphylococcal protein A[76,77]
Alteration of granulocyte functions	Opsonic assay[78-80]

(Reprinted with permission from Clay ME, Stroncek DF.[7])

and IgM complement-activating antibodies have been detected in patients with autoimmune neutropenia, febrile reactions and pulmonary transfusion reactions; many clinically important IgG antibodies cause agglutination but not complement activation.[66,82-85] In one study, there was no relationship between the Ig class or IgG subclass of granulocyte antibodies and the clinical effect of the antibody.[82]

Because of the nature of the clinical situation and the use of the agglutination assay, most antibodies involved in alloimmune neonatal neutropenia are IgG. Also, several studies in aggregate indicate that IgG antibodies are the most common type in autoimmune neutropenia.[84,85]

Alloantibodies vs Autoantibodies

Both allo- and autoantibodies to granulocyte-specific antigens occur. There is no immunochemical or serologic characteristic that distinguishes them. Both types of antibodies can be detected by leukoagglutination and may be of various immunoglobulin classes. Thus, when patients' sera are tested, there are no particular features that would suggest either auto- or allogeneic reactivity.

Drug-Related Granulocyte Antibodies

Granulocytopenia is a common side effect of many drugs. Most often this is due to the suppression of myelopoiesis; however, immune-mediated drug-related granulocytopenia may occur[86] (Table 3-5). Several methods have been used to detect granulocyte drug antibodies, making it difficult to compare the results of different studies and to conclude whether any particular antibody detection method is superior. Methods include agglutination, cytotoxicity, immunofluorescence, staphylococcal protein A, ELISA and immunoprecipitation. Most of these assays are done by including the drug in the assay system, but some drug antibodies react with metabolites of the drug,[100] or react best either when the drug is present or has been incubated but then washed away prior to the serum-cell incubation.

Sera containing drug-dependent antibodies may also react with other blood cells such as red cells or platelets.[7,94,101,105] Most granulocyte drug antibodies react with mature granulocytes, but some also react with immature granulocytes,[91,93,110,118] thus causing a suppression of myelopoiesis.

Cell Bound vs Serum Antibodies

In red blood cell serology, it is often important to determine not only whether antibody is present in the serum but also whether the

Table 3-5. Drugs Causing Immune-Mediated Neutropenia

Antiarrhythmias

Aprindine Hydrochloride[87]
Flecanide acetate[88]
Procainamide[89,90]
Quinidine[89,91–99]

Antibiotics

Ampicillin[96,97]
Amoxycillin[96]
Cephradine[98]
Cefotaxime[96,99]
Ceftazidime[96]
Cefuroxime[99]
Dicloxacillin[89]
Nafcillin[89]
Oxacillin[89,96]
Penicillin[96,100,101]
Sulfathiazole[102]
Sulphafurazole[89]

Antimalarial

Amodiaquine[103,104]
Chloroquine[102]
Quinine[105,106]

Analgesics and Anti-Inflammatory Agents

Aminopyrine[102,107,108]
Aminosalicylic acid[109]
Dicolofenac[100]
Dimethylaminophenazone[100]
Ibuprofen[110]
Propyphenazone[100]
Sulfapyridine[111]

Antithyroid

Propylthiouracil[101,112–117]
Carbimazole[113]
Methimazole[89,115,116]

Miscellaneous

Chloral hydrate[107]
Chloropropamide[118,119]
Clozapine[120]
Gold Thiomalate[101,102]
Levamisole[121,122]
Mercuhydrin[121]
Phenytoin[123,124]

(Reprinted with permission from Clay ME, Stroncek DF.[86])

antibody has bound to the cells. Only limited information of this sort is available for granulocytes. Elevated levels of IgG have been found on granulocytes from patients with primary autoimmune neutropenia, SLE and Felty's syndrome, but not on those from patients with several other diseases that appear to involve immune destruction of granulocytes. The techniques for detecting granulocyte-associated IgG are difficult. Also, in contrast to red cell autoimmune hemolytic anemia, there are often insufficient numbers of granulocytes to carry out a satisfactory test for cell-bound IgG. This assay is also complicated by the large number of Fc receptors on granulocytes with the resulting normal nonspecific binding of some IgG and/or immune complexes and the normal process of internalizing these. Thus, the determination of granulocyte-associated IgG has not been widely used.

Immune Complexes

Immune complexes bind to granulocytes through Fc and/or complement receptors and could theoretically be detected in some granulocyte antibody assays. There have been isolated reports of immune complexes in patients with Felty's syndrome, SLE and chronic idiopathic granulocytopenia[48]; however, immune complexes were not found in any of 29 patients with primary autoimmune neutropenia.[48] The role of immune complexes in the granulocytopenia of these immune diseases and in some granulocyte antibody tests remains to be finalized.

Clinical Situations Involving Alloantibodies

Neutropenia or granulocytopenia can be due to either production or increased destruction. For the most part, granulocyte alloantigen systems are involved in increased destruction, although some situations may appear to be decreased production if there is increased destruction of very immature myeloid precursors. This latter situation is not well understood, as very few studies have been done. For convenience, clinical situations involving alloantibodies will be distinguished from those involving autoantibodies.

Alloimmune Neonatal Neutropenia

In ANN, the mother is immunized to a granulocyte antigen that the fetus inherits from the father.[2] During pregnancy, maternal IgG granulocyte antibody crosses the placenta and destroys the fetus' granulocytes. However, since during gestation the fetus is protected from infections, the infant is asymptomatic at birth, but develops infection at a few days to weeks of life. It is estimated that ANN occurs as often as 2 in 1000 live births and in one study accounted for 1.5% of admissions to a neonatal intensive care unit and 16% of neutropenic patients with infection or sepsis.[125] Most infants experience only mild infections, including skin, urinary or respiratory tract, otitis or omphalitis.[3,126] The mortality from ANN is approximately 5%.[126] Treatment is with antibiotics and, if necessary, exchange transfusion to remove the offending antibody. Patients recover spontaneously in 2 weeks to 6 months as the maternal IgG is catabolized and the neutrophil count returns to normal. The antibodies most commonly involved in ANN are NA1 and NB1,[3,49] which are usually detected by agglutination techniques. Although some antibodies in ANN have been detected by other methods, no comprehensive study has been done to define the optimal technique for the diagnosis of ANN. One of the main problems in ANN is that differential leukocyte counts are not usually performed routinely and often the diagnosis is not considered initially. Thus, awareness of this situation is important as it can speed the diagnosis of the underlying cause of the neutropenia even when the infection is being properly treated.

Transfusion Reactions

It is well known that most febrile nonhemolytic transfusion reactions are due to leukocyte antibodies in the recipient, which react with leukocytes in the transfused blood component.[127,128] One unresolved issue is which antibody detection method best predicts a transfusion reaction. Leukoagglutination and lymphocytotoxicity are the methods most commonly used to detect leukocyte antibodies, but as many as one third of patients who develop febrile transfusion reactions do not have leukoagglutinins[129] and many patients who have lymphocytotoxic antibodies and receive a transfusion do not have febrile transfusion reactions.[130,131]

Typically, a febrile nonhemolytic reaction begins 30-60 minutes after the transfusion is begun. The patient experiences chills, general myalgia, headache, fever, flush palpitation, tachycardia, cough, irritability, confusion and dyspnea. The reaction may range from rather mild to severe. The degree of temperature increase is related to the number of leukocytes in the transfused component,[132] with fever being rare when fewer than 0.25×10^9 are given. These reactions are usually managed by switching the patient to leukocyte-depleted blood components after a reaction has occurred (rather than testing all potential transfusion recipients for leukocyte antibodies before transfusion) because the antibody detection methods are not sufficiently accurate to predict those patients who would have a reaction.

Some patients have a very severe form of nonhemolytic reaction that has been called transfusion-related acute lung injury (TRALI).[133] The reaction is similar to adult respiratory distress syndrome and is characterized by acute respiratory distress, bilateral pulmonary edema and severe hypoxemia. There may be associated fever and hypotension unresponsive to fluid administration. Although severe and dramatic, TRALI can be treated successfully if proper measures are taken. These include prompt aggressive respiratory support, such as intubation, and mechanical ventilation, if necessary, along with maintenance of blood pressure and diuresis. For a number of years, this syndrome was reported only occasionally and was thought to be a rare occurrence; however, reports have been increasing, probably due to improved recognition of the situation. In a recent review of published reports and personal experience, Popovsky et al[133] concluded that the common denominator in these reactions is plasma (in the form of whole blood, fresh frozen plasma, red cells stored in plasma or platelet concentrates). It appears that plasma containing leukocyte antibodies may be the inciting factor in these reactions.[4,133] Virtually all cases studied have involved the transfusion of plasma containing antibodies detected either by leukoagglutination, lymphocytotoxicity and, in many cases, the antibody had specificity against the recipient's cells for either HLA or neutrophil-specific antigens.[133] The pathophysiology by which transfusion of a relatively small amount of plasma containing antibody could cause such a severe systemic reaction is not clear. Popovsky et al[133] have suggested that activation of complement leading to granulocyte activation, release of toxic oxygen products, endothelial damage to the pulmonary vasculature and pulmonary edema might be involved. In order to prevent TRALI, they have proposed that plasma from multiparous donors not be used for transfusion unless it is known to be free of leukocyte antibodies.[133] This recommendation has not been adopted as yet. It remains important to be alert to the possibility of TRALI and to implement proper care quickly.

Granulocyte Transfusion

Granulocyte transfusions are seldom used today and, thus, the development of methods to match donor and recipient are not of high priority. If techniques become available to produce large numbers of granulocytes, causing a renewed interest in granulocyte transfusion, then renewed interest in granulocyte matching would follow.

Studies done when granulocyte transfusions were more widely used will be summarized here. Initially, it was believed that HLA compatibility between donor and recipient as determined by leukoagglutination or lymphocytotoxicity would be an effective way of matching for and providing an effective granulocyte transfusion and would improve the outcome.[134-136] However, other experience did not support this.[137] One problem with these studies was that several different leukocyte antibody detection methods were used and it was difficult to determine the fate of transfused granulocytes. Thus, careful studies correlating laboratory tests of compatibility with in-vivo results were difficult to conduct. In a series of studies using 111-indium-labeled granulocytes, incompatibility between donor and recipient in a leukoagglutinin crossmatch was associated with reduced intravascular recovery and survival of transfused cells, failure of transfused cells to localize at known sites of infection and abnormal sequestration of transfused cells in the lungs.[138] Mismatch of some HLA antigens also was associated with reduced intravascular recovery and survival, suggesting that the HLA system and lymphocytotoxicity might also be factors in compatibility testing for granulocyte transfusion.[138]

As these studies were nearing completion, the use of granulocytes declined and a practical system to match the donor and recipient was never developed. In the few centers that continued to provide granulocyte transfusions, the patient's serum is screened for HLA or granulocyte antibodies periodically and when antibodies develop, transfusions are often discontinued or HLA-matched or family donors are sought. If granulocyte transfusion should become practical in the future, it would be necessary to develop practical methodology to select compatible donors to avoid immune destruction of the transfused cells.

Bone Marrow Transplantation

Matching for bone marrow transplantation is based upon the HLA system, lymphocytotoxicity testing and mixed lymphocyte culture. It is well known that marrow incompatible for ABO antigens can be transplanted successfully[139] because of the absence of these blood group antigens on hematopoietic precursors.[139,140] Thus, while red cell blood group incompatibility may cause hematologic problems such as delayed hemolysis,[141] these antigens are not taken into consideration in matching for marrow transplantation. If granulocyte-specific antigens are present on hematopoietic precursors, these could interfere with successful engraftment if there are recipient antibodies present against donor marrow. However, this does not appear to be the case. Granulocyte-specific antigens are not detected on granulocytes until the myelocyte stage[3,142]; thus, antibodies against these antigens in marrow transplant recipients should not interfere with engraftment. This has been substantiated clinically; marrow from an NA1-positive donor has been engrafted successfully into a patient with circulating anti-NA1 at a titer of (1:64).[143] Subsequently, Stroncek et al[144] showed that marrow from a donor with NB1-positive granulocytes engrafted, but that the recovery of peripheral blood granulocytes was delayed. Thus, it appears that the presence of an antibody against granulocyte-specific antigens does not prevent engraftment, but can be expected to delay the appearance of mature neutrophils in the circulation. This expected situation is analogous to the delayed reticulocytosis in recipients of ABO-incompatible marrow, which improves when the red cell antibody disappears.

Clinical Situations Involving Autoantibodies

Primary Autoimmune Neutropenia

Isolated neutropenia due to accelerated destruction occurs in both adults and children as an isolated hematologic abnormality, with no associated diseases or factors that might account for the neutropenia. The destruction is immunologic and frequently these patients have granulocyte antibodies. Lalezari[145] and Boxer[146] showed that, in these patients, antineutrophil antibodies were present and reacted with the patient's own neutrophils; upon their disappearance, the neutrophil count returned to normal. A number of more recent studies have documented similar cases. Autoimmune neutropenia has been best described in children.[66,83,146-161] The onset of neutropenia has occurred at 3-30 months of age, with a median of about 8 months.[4,145,162] The neutrophil level returns to normal spontaneously, with a median duration of neutropenia of 13-20 months.[4,145,162] Usually, the patients present with fever and infections involving the skin, otitis media, respiratory tract and/or urinary tract. Life-threatening infections are rare. The neutrophil count is usually less than $500/\mu L$,[145-162] and the bone marrow is normal to hypercellular, with a decrease in more mature myeloid elements so that the marrow has the appearance of a "maturation arrest" at the metamyelocyte stage.[4] Maturation arrest is a misnomer, however, since the situation is really an accelerated destruction of more mature forms. In fact, the more the patient's serum reacts with immature myeloid forms, the more severe the neutropenia. Treatment should be directed toward the infection. Steroids are not usually effective.[145] Intravenous immune globulin has provided transient increases in the neutrophil count and two of eight patients had a complete remission.[145,163]

Antibodies to granulocytes have been demonstrated in virtually all of these patients,[4,85,145,162] the most common specificity being NA1, which has been found in 10-46% of patients.[85,145,162] In our experience with 36 of these patients, anti-NA1 was found in all of 17 patients in whom the antibody had specificity. No extensive studies have compared the effectiveness of different leukocyte antibody detection methods for the diagnosis of autoimmune neutropenia. Since leukoagglutination is the most commonly used test, most patients have been found to have agglutinating antibodies.[4] Very few of our patients had HLA or lymphocytotoxic antibodies. The granulocyte antibodies are usually IgG, although we did not find a relationship between the Ig class of the antibody and the strength of reactivity in different assays or the patients' clinical course.[4]

Although neutropenia may occur as an isolated or primary autoimmune event in adults, it is more commonly associated with other immunologic abnormalities or malignancy and, thus, is referred to as secondary autoimmune neutropenia.[85]

Secondary Autoimmune Neutropenia

Granulocytopenia is a common feature of many autoimmune diseases. The pathophysiology is often not known, but could involve immune complexes, complement activation or formation of antibodies that crossreact with granulocytes. Granulocyte antibodies occur in several immunologic or malignant diseases where it appears that the antibodies are a part of a broader immunologic abnormality and seem to be responsible for the observed neutropenia. Thus, detection of these autoantibodies can be of assistance in determining the cause of the neutropenia. Unfortunately, in many of these clinical situations, granulocyte antibodies have not been detected. A variety of methods has been used to detect these autoantibodies.[48] Some methods are more effective in particular clinical situations, although, in many cases, multiple methods have not been compared so the optimal method may not be known and the method originally reported for that clinical situation is used.

Autoimmune neutropenia in association with several vasculitis-type diseases in which anticytoplasmic antibodies are present has been discussed earlier. There are a number of other diseases in which secondary autoimmune neutropenia occurs. The most common of these are: autoimmune hemolytic anemia, SLE, Felty's syndrome, infectious mononucleosis, lymphatic malignancy, immune deficiency diseases, thyroid diseases and scleroderma.[4,7] Severe or life-threatening infections are not usual in these patients, and the therapy is directed toward the underlying disease and the specific infection when one occurs. A few patients have been treated with steroids, intravenous immune globulin or granulocyte/macrophage colony-stimulating factor, with transient improvement in granulocyte count.[164-169]

A number of patients with T lymphocytosis and neutropenia have been reported. In general, these patients with an expanded T-cell population have an increased number of T cells of the T8 or suppressor type, which are large granular lymphocytes.[170,171] Some patients have increased neutrophil-associated IgG and shortened intravascular half-life, while others demonstrate cytotoxicity of marrow progenitors or production of inhibitory cytokines.[170,172] In some patients, this syndrome is chronic and benign, lasting for 20 years. The patients experience infections of the skin and oropharynx, although these are not usually serious. In other patients, the syndrome involves a malignant transformation of the lymphocytes and, in one recent report, the lymphocytes were infected with HTLV-II.[173]

A more extensive list of the diseases associated with autoimmune neutropenia is provided in Table 3-6.

Conclusions

Granulocyte-specific antigens and antibodies are important and of interest because they are involved in clinical situations such as immune neutropenia and transfusion reactions and because the antigens are being increasingly recognized as part of molecules that have important functions in or on the granulocyte membrane. Although clinical testing for granulocyte antibodies is not a high-volume activity, it is important that the transfusion medicine community continue to investigate these antigens and antibodies in order to better understand granulocyte structure and function and their role in clinical practice.

Table 3-6. Diseases Associated With Secondary Autoimmune Granulocytopenia

Autoimmune Disorders

Rheumatoid arthritis[85,174,175]
Felty's syndrome[85,174,176]
Systemic lupus erythematosus[85,174,175,176]
Sjögren's disease[164,174]
Mixed connective tissue syndrome[84]
Polymyalgia rheumatica[85]
Hashimoto's thyroiditis[174,175]
Immune-complex glomerulonephritis[174]
Wegener's granulomatosis[85]
Primary biliary cirrhosis[85,177]
Myasthenia gravis[164,174]

Autoimmune Hematologic Disorders

Autoimmune thrombocytopenia[85,164,174]
Autoimmune hemolytic anemia[84,164]
Autoimmune thrombocytopenia and hemolytic anemia
    (Evan's syndrome)[85,164,174]

Hematologic Malignancies

Leukemia[85]
Hodgkin's disease[85]
Non-Hodgkin's lymphoma[85]

Immune Deficiencies

HIV infection[85,178]
Common variable immune deficiency[85]

Other

Myelodysplastic syndrome[175]
Crohn's disease[175]
Acute rheumatic fever[174]

(Reprinted with permission from Clay ME, Stroncek DF.[7])

References

1. Doan CA. The recognition of a biologic differentiation in the white blood cells. JAMA 1926;86;21:1593-7.
2. Lalezari P, Nussbaum M, Gelman S, Spaet TH. Neonatal neutropenia due to maternal isoimmunization. Blood 1960;14:236-42.
3. Lalezari P, Radel E. Neutrophil-specific antigens: Immunology and clinical significance. Semin Hematol 1974;11:281-90.
4. McCullough J. The clinical significance of granulocyte antibodies and in vivo studies of the fate of granulocytes. In: Garratty G, ed. Current concepts in transfusion therapy. Arlington, VA: American Association of Blood Banks, 1985:125-81.
5. Otho H, Matsuo Y. Neutrophil-specific antigens and gene frequencies in Japanese. Transfusion 1989;29:654-63.
6. Schnell M, Halligan G, Herman J. A new granulocyte antibody directed at a high frequency antigen causing neonatal alloimmune neutropenia (abstract). Transfusion 1989;29:46S.
7. Clay ME, Stroncek DF. Granulocyte immunology. In: Ness P, Anderson K, eds. Scientific basis of transfusion medicine. Philadelphia: WB Saunders, 1993 (in press).
8. Werner G, von dem Borne AEGKr, Bos MJE, et al. Localization of human NA1 alloantigen on neutrophil Fc receptors. In: Reinherz EL, Haynes BF, Nadler LM, Bernstein ID, eds. Leukocyte typing II: Human myeloid and hematopoietic cells. New York: Springer-Verlag, 1986:109-21.
9. Huizinga TWJ, Kleijer M, Tetteroo PAT, et al. Biallelic neutrophil NA-antigen system is associated with a polymorphism on the phosphoinositol-linked Fc-receptor III (CD16). Blood 1990;75:213-7.
10. Huizinga TWJ, Juijpers RWAM, Kleijer M, et al. Maternal genomic neutrophil FcRIII deficiency leading to neonatal isoimmune neutropenia. Blood 1990;76:1927-32.
11. Huizinga TWJ, de Haas M, Kleijer M, et al. Soluble Fc receptor III in human plasma originated from release by neutrophils. J Clin Invest 1990;86:416-23.
12. Stroncek DF, Skubitz KM, McCullough JJ. Biochemical characterization of the neutrophil-specific antigen NB1. Blood 1990; 75:744-55.
13. Goldschmeding R, van Dalen CM, Faber N, et al. Further characterization of the NB1 antigen as a variably expressed 56-65 kDa GPI-linked glycoprotein of plasma membranes and specific granules of neutrophils. Br J Haematol 1992;81:336-45.
14. Skubitz KM, Stroncek DF, Sun B. The neutrophil-specific antigen NB1 is anchored via a glycosyl-phosphatidylinositol linkage. J Leukoc Biol 1991;49:163-71.

15. Trounstine ML, Peitz GA, Yssel H, et al. Reactivity of cloned, expressed human FcRIII isoforms with monoclonal antibodies which distinguish cell type specific and allelic forms of Fc-gamma-RIII. Int Immunol 1990;2:303-10.

16. Ory PA, Clark MR, Kwoh EE, et al. Sequences of complementary DNAs that encode the NA1 and NA2 forms of Fc receptor on human neutrophils. J Clin Invest 1989;84:1688-91.

17. Faber V, Elling P, Norup G, et al. An antinuclear factor specific for leukocytes. Lancet 1974;2:344-5.

18. Wiik A, Munthe E. Restriction among heavy and light chain determinants of granulocyte-specific antinuclear factors. Immunology 1972;23:53-60.

19. van der Woude FJ, Rasmussen N, Lobatto S, et al. Autoantibodies against neutrophils and monocytes: Tool for diagnosis and marker of disease activity in Wegener's granulomatosis. Lancet 1985;1:425-9.

20. Rasmussen N, Wiik A. Autoimmunity in Wegener's granulomatoses. Immunobiology autoimmunity and transplantation in otorhinolaryngology. In: Veldman JE, McCabe BF, Houzing EH, Mygind N, eds. Proceedings of the 1st International Conference. Utrecht, The Netherlands, 1984. Amsterdam: Kugler Publications, 1984:231-6.

21. Kallenberg CGM, Mulder AHL, Tervaert JWC. Antineutrophil cytoplasmic antibodies: A still-growing class of autoantibodies in inflammatory disorders. Am J Med 1992;93:675-82.

22. Salmon JE, Edberg JC, Kimberly RP. Fcγ receptor III on human neutrophils: Allelic variants have functionally distinct capacities. J Clin Invest 1990;85:1287-95.

23. Knapp W, Dorken B, Rieber P, et al. CD antigens 1989. Blood 1980;74:1448-50.

24. Huizinga TWJ, Kleijer M, Roos D, von dem Borne AEGKr. Differences between FcRIII of human neutrophils and human K/NK lymphocytes in relation to the NA antigen system. In: Knapp W, Dorken B, Gilks SR, et al, eds. Leucocyte typing IV. White cell differentiation antigens. Oxford: Oxford University Press, 1989:582-5.

25. Hogs N, Horton MA. Myeloid antigens: New and previously defined clusters. In: McMichael AJ, ed. Leucocyte typing III. White cell differentiation antigens. Oxford: Oxford University Press, 1989:576-602.

26. Clement LT, Lehmeyer JE, Gartland GL. Identification of neutrophil subpopulations with monoclonal antibodies. Blood 1983;61:326-32.

27. Ahearn JM, Fearon DT. Structure and function of the complement receptors, CR1 (CD35) and CR2 (CD21). Adv Immunol 1989;46:183-219.

28. Kishimoto TK, Larson RS, Corbi AL, et al. The leukocyte integrins. Adv Immunol 1989;46:149-82.
29. Boulay F, Tardif M, Brouchon L, Vignais P. The human N-formylpeptide receptor. Characterization of two cDNA isolates and evidence for a new subfamily of G-protein coupled receptors. Biochemistry 1990;29:11123-33.
30. Gerard NP, Gerard C. The chemotactic receptor for human C5a anaphylatoxin. Nature 1991;349:614-17.
31. Murphy PM, Tiffany HL. Cloning of complementary DNA encoding a functional human interleukin-8 receptor. Science 1991; 253:1280-3.
32. Ruosalahti E. Integrins. J Clin Invest 1991;87:1-5.
33. Anderson DC, Springer TA. Leukocyte adhesion deficiency: An inherited defect in Mac-1, LFA-1, and p150, 95 glycoproteins. Annu Rev Med 1987;38:175-94.
34. Etzioni A, Frydman M, Pollack S, et al. Brief report: Recurrent severe infections caused by a novel leukocyte adhesion deficiency. N Engl J Med 1992;327:1789-92.
35. Albelda SM, Buck CA. Integrins and other cell adhesion molecules. FASEB J 1990;4:2868-80.
36. Wright SD, Detmers PA. Adhesion-promoting receptors on phagocytes. J Cell Sci Suppl 1988;9:99-120.
37. Kappelmayer J, Bernabei A, Gikakis N, et al. Upregulation of Mac-1 surface expression on neutrophils during simulated extracorporeal circulation. J Lab Clin Med 1993;121:118-26.
38. Springer TA, Lasky LA. Sticky sugars for selectins. Nature 1991;349:196-7.
39. Larsen GR, Sako D, Ahern JM, et al. P-selectin and E-selectin: Distinct but overlapping leukocyte ligand specificities. J Biol Chem 1992;267:11104-41.
40. Bevilacqua MP, Nelsen RV. Selectins. J Clin Invest 1993;91:379-87.
41. Gallatin WM, Weisman IL, Butcher EC. A cell surface molecule involved in organ-specific homing of lymphocytes. Nature 1983; 304:30-4.
42. Griffin JD, Spertini O, Ernst TJ, et al. Granulocyte-macrophage colony-stimulating factor and other cytokines regulate surface expression of the leukocyte adhesion molecule-1 on human neutrophils, monocytes and their precursors. J Immunol 1990; 145:576-84.
43. Jutila MA, Kishimoto TK, Butcher EC. Regulation and selectin activity of the human neutrophil peripheral lymph node homing receptor. Blood 1990;76:178-83.
44. Spertini O, Kansas GS, Munro M, et al. Regulation of leukocyte migration by activation of the leukocyte adhesion molecule-1 (LAM-1) selectin. Nature 1991;349:691-4.

45. Clark MR, Liu L, Clarkson SB, et al. An abnormality of the gene that encodes neutrophil Fc receptor III in a patient with systemic lupus erythematosus. J Clin Invest 1990;86:341-6.
46. van der Schoot CE, Daams M, Hiskes E, et al. Antigenic polymorphism of the Leu-CAM family recognized by human leukocyte alloantisera. Br J Haematol 1993 (in press).
47. Richards KL, McCullough J. Association between NB1 neutrophil-specific antigen and FMLP chemotaxis (abstract). J Cell Biol 1984;99:279a.
48. Clay ME, Kline WE. Detection of granulocyte antigens and antibodies. Current perspectives and approaches. In: Garratty G, ed. Current concepts in transfusion therapy. Arlington, VA: American Association of Blood Banks, 1984:183-265.
49. McCullough J, Press C, Clay M, Cline W. Granulocyte serology. Chicago, IL: American Society of Clinical Pathologists, 1988.
50. Lalezari P, Bernard GE. Improved leukocyte antibody detection with prolonged incubation. Vox Sang 1964;9:664-72.
51. Lalezari P, Jiange A, Lee S. A microagglutination technique for detection of leukocyte agglutinins. In: Ray JG, Hare DB, Pederson PD, Mallally DI, eds. NIAID manual of tissue typing techniques. DHEW Publication # (NIH) 77-545. Washington, DC: US Government Printing Office, 1976-77:4-6.
52. Lalezari P, Pryce SC. Detection of neutrophil and platelet antibodies in immunologically induced neutropenia and thrombocytopenia. In: Rose NR, Friedmann H, eds. Manual of clinical immunology. Washington, DC: American Society for Microbiology 1980:744-9.
53. Thompson JS, Severson CD, Lavender AR, et al. Assay of human leukoagglutinins by capillary migration. Transplantation 1968; 6:728-36.
54. Severson CD, Greazel NA, Thompson JS. Micro-capillary agglutination. J Immunol Methods 1974;4:369-80.
55. McCullough J, Burke ME, Wood N, et al. Microcapillary agglutination for the detection of leukocyte antibodies: Evaluation of the method and clinical significance in transfusion reactions. Transfusion 1974;14:425-32.
56. Hasegawa T, Graw RG, Terasaki PI. A microgranulocyte cytotoxicity test. Transplantation 1974;15:492-8.
57. Caplan SN, Berkman EM, Babior BM. Cytotoxins against a granulocyte antigen system: Detection by a new method employing cytochalasin-B-treated cells. Vox Sang 1977;33:206-11.
58. Drew SI, Bergh O, McClelland J, et al. Antigenic specificities detected on papainized human granulocytes by microgranulocytotoxicity. Transplant Proc 1977;9:639-45.
59. Drew SI, Carter BM, Guidera D, et al. Further aspects of microgranulocytotoxicity. Transfusion 1979;19:434-43.

60. Hasegawa T, Bergh OJ, Mickey MR, Terasaki PI. Preliminary human granulocyte specificities. Transplant Proc 1975;7:75-80.
61. Takasugi M. Improved fluorochromatic cytotoxic test. Transplantation 1971;12:148-51.
62. Engelfriet CP, Tetteroo PAT, van der Veen JPW, et al. Granulocyte-specific antigens and methods for their detection. In: McCullough J, Sandler SG, eds. Advances in immunobiology: Blood cell antigens and bone marrow transplantation. New York: Alan R. Liss, 1984:121-54.
63. Logue GL, Kurlander R, Pepe P, et al. Antibody-dependent lymphocyte-mediated granulocyte cytotoxicity in man. Blood 1978;51:97-108.
64. Richards K, Sadrzadeh SMH, Clay M, McCullough J. Antibody-dependent lymphocyte-mediated granulocytotoxicity (ADLG) for the detection of granulocyte antibodies. J Immunol Methods 1983;63:93-102.
65. Verheugt FWA, von dem Borne AEGKr, Decary S, et al. The detection of granulocyte alloantibodies with an indirect immunofluorescence test. Br J Haematol 1977;36:533-44.
66. Verheugt FWA, von dem Borne AEGKr, van Noord-Bokhorst JC, et al. Autoimmune granulocytopenia: The detection of granulocyte autoantibodies with the immunofluorescence test. Br J Haematol 1978;39:339-50.
67. von dem Borne AEGKr, van dem Plas-van Dalen C, Engelfriet CP. Immunofluorescence antiglobulin test. In: McMillan R, ed. Immune cytopenias. New York: Churchill Livingstone, 1983: 106-27.
68. Zaroulis CG, Jaramillo S. A microimmunofluorescent assay to detect human granulocyte antigens and antibodies. Am J Hematol 1981;10:65-73.
69. Press C, Kline WE, Clay ME, McCullough J. A microtiter modification of granulocyte immunofluorescence. Vox Sang 1985;49:110-13.
70. Lalezari P, Khorshidi M. Detection of neutrophil and platelet antibodies: Agglutination, immunofluorscence and flow cytometry. In: Greenwalt TJ, ed. Blood transfusion: Methods in hematology. New York: Churchill Livingstone, 1988: 149-62.
71. Henke M, Yonemoto LM, Lazar GS, et al. Visual detection of granulocyte surface antigens using the avidin-biotin complex. J Histochem Cytochem 1984;32:712-16.
72. Mannoni P, Janowska-Wieczorek A, Turner AR, et al. Monoclonal antibodies against human granulocytes and myeloid differentiation antigens. Hum Immunol 1982;5:309-23.
73. Braman AM, Davis J, Schwartz KA. A radioimmune microfilter plate assay for the detection of anti-granulocyte antibodies (abstract). Blood 1991;78(Suppl 1):347a.

74. Rustagi PK, Currie MS, Logue GL. Complement-activating anti-neutrophil antibody in systemic lupus erythematosus. Am J Med 1985;78:971-7.
75. Cines DB, Pessaro F, Guerry D, et al. Granulocyte-associated IgG in neutropenic disorders. Blood 1982;59:124-32.
76. McCallister JA, Boxer LA, Baehner RL. The use and limitation of labeled staphylococcal protein A for study of antineutrophil antibodies. Blood 1979;54:1330-7.
77. Lazar GS, Gaidulis L, Henke M, Blume KG. A sensitive screening method of detecting anti-granulocyte antibodies employing radio labeled staphylococcal protein A. J Immunol Methods 1984;68:1-9.
78. Boxer LA, Stossel TP. Effects of anti-human neutrophil antibodies in vitro. Quantitative studies. J Clin Invest 1974;53:1534-45.
79. Boxer LA, Greenberg SM, Boxer GJ, Stossel SP. Autoimmune neutropenia. N Engl J Med 1975;293:748-53.
80. Drew S, Terasaki PI. Autoimmune cytotoxic granulocyte antibodies in normal persons and various diseases. Blood 1978;52:941-52.
81. Thompson JS, Overlin VL, Herbick JM, et al. New granulocyte antigens demonstrated by microgranulocytotoxicity assay. J Clin Invest 1980;65:1431-9.
82. Verheugt FWA, von dem Borne AEGKr, van Noord-Bokhorst JC, et al. Serological immunochemical and immunocytological properties of granulocyte antibodies. Vox Sang 1978;35:294-303.
83. McCullough J, Clay ME, Priest JR, et al. A comparison of methods for detecting leukocyte antibodies in autoimmune neutropenia. Transfusion 1981;21:483-92.
84. Bux J, Jung KD, Kauth T, Mueller-Eckhardt C. Serological and clinical aspects of granulocyte antibodies leading to alloimmune neonatal neutropenia. Transfus Med 1992;2:143-59.
85. Bux J, Kissel K, Nowak K, et al. Autoimmune neutropenia: Clinical and laboratory studies in 143 patients. Ann Hematol 1991;63:243-52.
86. Stroncek DF. Drug-induced immune neutropenia. Transfus Med Rev 1993 (in press).
87. Pisciotta AV, Cronkite C. Aprindine-induced agranulocytosis: Evidence for immunologic mechanism. Arch Intern Med 1983;143:241-3.
88. Samlowski WE, Frame RN, Logue GL. Flecanide-induced immune neutropenia. Documentation of a hepten-mediated mechanism of cell destruction. Arch Intern Med 1987;147:383-4.
89. Weitzman SA, Stossel TP, Desmond M. Drug-induced immunological neutropenia. Lancet 1978;1:1068-72.

90. Yomtovian R, Kline W, Press C, et al. Evidence for granulocyte antibody activity in two cases of procainamide-associated neutropenia (abstract). Blood 1984;64:92a.
91. Kelton JG, Huang AT, Mold N, et al. The use of in vitro techniques to study drug-induced pancytopenia. N Engl J Med 1979;301:621-4.
92. Eisner EV, Carr RV, MacKinney AA. Quinidine-induced agranulocytosis. JAMA 1977;238:884-6.
93. Ascensao JL, Flynn PJ, Slungaard A, et al. Quinidine-induced neutropenia: Report of a case with drug-dependent inhibition of granulocyte colony generation. Acta Haematol 1984;72:349-54.
94. Chong BH, Berndt ME, Koutts J, et al. Quinidine-induced thrombocytopenia and leukopenia: Demonstration and characterization of distinct antiplatelet and antileukocyte antibodies. Blood 1983;62:1218-23.
95. Alexander SJ, Gilmore RI. Quinidine-induced agranulocytosis. Am J Hematol 1984;16:95-8.
96. Rouveix B, Lassoued K, Vittecoq D, et al. Neutropenia due to β lactam antibodies. Br Med J 1983;287:1832-4.
97. Pisciotta AV. Agranulocytosis during antibiotic therapy: Drug sensitivity or sepsis? Am J Hematol 1993;42:132-7.
98. Lawson AA, McArdle T, Ghosh S. Cephadrine-associated immune neutropenia (letter). N Engl J Med 1985;312:651.
99. Murphy MF, Metcalfe PC, Grint PCA, et al. Cephalosporin-induced immune neutropenia. Br J Haematol 1985;59:9-14.
100. Salama A, Schutz B, Kiefel V, et al. Immune-mediated agranulocytosis related to drugs and their metabolites: Mode of sensitization and heterogeneity of antibodies. Br J Haematol 1989;72:127-32.
101. Murphy MF, Riordan T, Minchinton RV, et al. Demonstration of an immune-mediated mechanism of penicillin-induced neutropenia and thrombocytopenia. Br J Haematol 1983;55:155-60.
102. Tullis JT. Prevalence, nature and identification of leukocyte antibodies. N Engl J Med 1958;258:569-78.
103. Rouveix B, Coulombel L, Aymard JP, et al. Amodiaquine-induced immune agranulocytosis. Br J Haematol 1989;75:7-11.
104. Douer D, Schwartz E, Shaked N, et al. Amodiaquine-induced agranulocytosis: Drug inhibition of myeloid colonies in the presence of patient's serum. Isr J Med Sci 1985;21:331-4.
105. Stroncek DF, Vercellotti GM, Hammerschmidt DE, et al. Characterization of multiple quinine-dependent antibodies in a patient with episodic hemolytic uremic syndrome and immune agranulocytosis. Blood 1992;80:241-8.
106. Maguire RB, Stroncek DF, Cambell AC. Recurrent pancytopenia, coagulopathy, and renal failure associated with multiple

quinine-dependent antibodies. Ann Intern Med 1993;119:215-17.
107. Tullis JL. The role of leukocyte and platelet antibody tests in the management of diverse clinical disorders. Ann Intern Med 1961;64:1165-80.
108. Moeschlin S, Wagner K. Agranulocytosis due to the occurrence of leukocyte-agglutinins. Acta Haematol 1952;8:29-51.
109. Dausset J, Bergerot-Blondel Y. Étude d'un anticorps allergique actif en présence de para-amino-salicylate de soude (PAS) contre les hématies, les leukocytes et les plaquettes humaines. Vox Sang 1961;6:91-109.
110. Mamus SW, Burton JD, Groat JD, et al. Ibuprofen-associated pure white-cell aplasia. N Engl J Med 1986;314:624-5.
111. Moeschlin S. Immunological granulocytopenia and agranulo-cytosis. Sang 1955;26:32-51.
112. Berkman EM, Orlin JB, Wolfsdorf J. An anti-neutrophil antibody associated with a propylthiouracil-induced lupus-like syndrome. Transfusion 1983;23:135-8.
113. Fibbe WE, Claas FHJ, van der Star-Dijkstra W, et al. Agranulo-cytosis induced by propylthiouracil: Evidence of a drug-dependent antibody reacting with granulocytes, monocytes and haematopoietic progenitor cells. Br J Haematol 1986;64:363-73.
114. Sato K, Miyakawa M, Han DC, et al. Graves' disease with neutropenia and marked splenomegaly: Autoimmune neu-tropenia due to propylthiouracil. J Endocrinol Invest 1985;8:551-5.
115. Wall JR, Fang SL, Kuroki T, et al. In vitro immunoreactivity to propylthiouracil, methimazole, and carbimazole in patients with Graves' disease: A possible cause of antithyroid drug-induced agranulocytosis. J Clin Endocrinol Metab 1984;58:868-72.
116. Bilezikian SB, Laleli Y, Tsan MF, et al. Immunological reactions involving leukocytes: III. Agranulocytosis induced by antithy-roid drugs. Johns Hopkins Med J 1976;138:124-9.
117. Guffy MM, Goeken NE, Burns CP. Granulocytotoxic antibodies in a patient with propylthiouracil induced agranulocytosis. Arch Intern Med 1984;144:1687-8.
118. Levitt LJ. Chloropropamide-induced pure white cell aplasia. Blood 1987;69:394-400.
119. Stein JH, Hamilton HE, Sheefs RF. Agranulocytosis caused by chloropropamide. Arch Intern Med 1964;113:78-82.
120. Pisciottta AV, Konings SA, Ciespmier LL, et al. Cytotoxic activity in serum of patients with clozapine-induced agranulocyto-sis. J Lab Clin Med 1992;119:254-66.
121. Thompson JS, Herbick JM, Klassen LW, et al. Studies on levamisole-induced agranulocytosis. Blood 1980;56:388-96.

122. Drew SI, Carter BM, Nathanson DS, et al. Levamisole-associated neutropenia and autoimmune granulocytotoxins. Ann Rheum Dis 1980;39:59-63.
123. Taetle R, Lane TA, Mendelsohn J. Drug-induced agranulocytosis: In vitro evidence for immune suppression of granulopoiesis and a cross-reacting lymphocyte antibody. Blood 1979;54:501-12.
124. Menitove JE, Rassiga AL, McLaren GD, et al. Antigranulocyte antibodies and deranged immune function associated with phenytoin-induced serum sickness. Am J Hematol 1981;10:277-84.
125. Levine DH, Madyastha PR, Wade TR, Levkoff AH. Isoimmnune neonatal neutropenia. Am J Perinatol 1987;3:231-3.
126. Lalezari P. Alloimmune neonatal neutropenia. In: Engelfriet CP, van Logham JJ, von dem Borne AEGKr, eds. Immunuhaematology. Amsterdam: Elsevier Science Publishers, 1984:179-86.
127. Brittingham TE, Chaplin H. Febrile transfusion reactions caused by sensitivity to donor leukocytes and platelets. JAMA 1947;165:819-25.
128. Payne R. The association of febrile transfusion reactions with leukoagglutinins. Vox Sang 1957;2:23341.
129. Payne R, Rolfs MR. Further observations on leukoagglutinin transfusion reactions. Am J Med 1960;29:449-58.
130. Decary F, Ferner P, Giavedoni L, et al. An investigation of nonhemolytic transfusion reactions. Vox Sang 1984;46:277-85.
131. de Rie MA, van der Plas-van Dorlen CM, Engelfriet CP, von dem Borne AEGKr. The serology of febrile transfusion reactions. Vox Sang 1985;49:126-34.
132. Perkins HA, Payne R, Ferguson J, Wood M. Non-hemolytic febrile transfusion reactions. Quantitative effects of blood components with emphasis on isoantigenic incompatibility of leukocytes. Vox Sang 1966;11:578-600.
133. Popovsky MA, Chaplin HC, Moore SB. Transfusion-related acute lung injury: A neglected, serious complication of hemotherapy. Transfusion 1992;32:589-92.
134. Graw RG, Herzig G, Perry S, Henderson ES. Normal granulocyte transfusion therapy. Treatment of septicemia due to gram-negative bacteria. N Engl J Med 1972;287:367-71.
135. Goldstein JM, Eyre HJ, Terasaki PI, et al. Leukocyte transfusions: Role of leukocyte alloantibodies in determining transfusion response. Transfusion 1971;11:19-24.
136. Graw RJ Jr, Stout FG, Herzig RH, Herzig GP. Granulocyte transfusion trials at the National Cancer Institute in the granulocyte: Function and clinical utilization. In: Greenwalt TJ, Jamieson GA, eds. Progress in clinical and biological research. New York: Alan R. Liss, Inc., 1977:267-81.

137. Dahlke MB, Keashen M, Alavi JB, et al. Granulocyte transfusion and outcome of alloimmunized patients with gram-negative sepsis. Transfusion 1982:22;374-81.

138. McCullough J, Clay M, Hurd D, et al. Effect of leukocyte antibodies and HLA matching on the intravascular recovery, survival, and tissue localization of 111-indium granulocytes. Blood 1986;67:522-8.

139. Warkentin PI, Hilden JM, Kersey JH, et al. Transplantation of major ABO-incompatible bone marrow depleted of red cells by hydroxyethyl starch. Vox Sang 1985;48:89-104.

140. Hershko C, Gale RP, Ho W, Fitchen J. ABH antigens and bone marrow transplantation. Br J Haematol 1980;44:65-73.

141. Warkentin P, Yomtovian R, Hurd D, et al. Severe delayed hemolytic transfusion reaction complicating an ABO-incompatible bone marrow transplantation. Vox Sang 1983;45:40-7.

142. Boxer LA, Yokoyama M, Lalezari P. Isoimmune neonatal neutropenia J Pediatr 1972;80:783-7.

143. Warkentin PI, Clay ME, Kersey JH, et al. Successful engraftment of NA1 positive bone marrow in a patient with the neutrophil antibody, anti-NA1. Hum Immunol 1981;2:173-84.

144. Stroncek DF, Shapiro R, Filipovich A, et al. Prolonged neutropenia following marrow transplant due to antibodies to neutrophil-specific antigen NB1. Transfusion 1993;33:158-63.

145. Lalezari P, Khorshidi M, Petrosova M. Autoimmune neutropenia of infancy. J Pediatr 1986;109:764-9.

146. Boxer LA, Greenberg S, Boxer GJ, Stossel TP. Autoimmune neutropenia. N Engl J Med 1975;293:748-53.

147. Lalezari P, Jiang A, Yegen L, Santorineou M. Chronic autoimmune neutropenia due to anti-NA2 antibody. N Engl J Med 1975;293:744-7.

148. Valbonesi M, Campelli A, Marazzi MG, et al. Chronic autoimmune neutropenia due to anti-NA1 antibody. Vox Sang 1979; 36:9-12.

149. Lightsey AL, Chapman RV, McMillan R, et al. Immune neutropenia. Ann Intern Med 1977;86:60-2.

150. Cline MJ, Opelz G, Saxon A, et al. Autoimmune panleukopenia. N Engl J Med 1976;295:1489-93.

151. Claas FHJ, Langerak J, Sabbe LJM, et al. NE1, a new neutrophil specific antigen. Tissue Antigens 1979;13:129-34.

152. Thompson BS, Darlow B, Stableforth P, et al. Auto-immune neutropenia in an infant. Postgrad Med J 1978;54:278-80.

153. Nepo AG, Gunay U, Boxer LA, et al. Autoimmune neutropenia in an infant. J Pediatr 1975;87:251-4.

154. Madyastha PR, Kyong CU, Darby CP, et al. Role of neutrophil antibody NA1 in an infant with autoimmune neutropenia. Am J Dis Child 1982;136:718-21.

155. Kay AB, White AG, Barclay GR, et al. Leukocyte function in a case of chronic benign neutropenia of infancy associated with circulating leukoagglutinins. Br J Haematol 1976;32:451-7.
156. Smith WK, Mold JW, Tseng SL, et al. Microcapillary agglutination assay for detection of specific antileukocyte reactivity in neutropenic patients. Am J Hematol 1979;7:329-40.
157. Bom-van Noorloos AA, Pegels HG, van Oers RHJ, et al. Proliferation of T cells with killer-cell activity in two patients with neutropenia and recurrent infections. N Engl J Med 1980;302:933-7.
158. Caligaris-Cappio F, Camussi G, Gavisto F. Idiopathic neutropenia with normal cellular bone marrow: An immune-complex disease. Br J Haematol 1979;43:595-605.
159. Carmel R. An unusual case of autoimmune agranulocytosis with total absence of myeloid precursors: Demonstration of diverse sources of R binder for Cobalamin in plasma and secretions. Am J Clin Pathol 1983;79:611-5.
160. Sabbe LJM, Claas FHJ, Langerak J, et al. Group-specific autoimmune antibodies directed to granulocytes as a cause of chronic benign neutropenia in infants. Acta Haematol 1982;68:20-7.
161. Freed N. Idiopathic autoimmune neutropenia. Report of a case. J Am Osteopath Assoc 1983;82:419-25.
162. Conway LT, Clay ME, Kline WE, et al. Natural history of primary autoimmune neutropenia in infancy. Pediatrics 1987;79:728-33.
163. Bussel J, Lalezari P, Fibrig S. Intravenous treatment with gammaglobulin of autoimmune neutropenia of infancy. J Pediatr 1988;112:298-301.
164. Beatty PA, Stroncek DF. Autoimmune neutropenia in Sheboygan County, Wisconsin. J Lab Clin Med 1992;119:718-23.
165. Gasner A, Ottmann OG, Erdmann H, et al. The effect of recombinant human granulocyte-macrophage colony-stimulating factor on neutropenia and related morbidity in chronic severe neutropenia. Ann Intern Med 1989;111:887-91.
166. Pollack S, Cunningham-Rundles C, Smithwick EM, et al. High-dose intravenous gamma globulin for autoimmune neutropenia (letter). N Engl J Med 1982;307:253.
167. Ricevuti G, Mazzone A, Rizzo SC. A study of neutrophil function in a case of associated autoimmune neutropenia and thrombocytopenia treated with high doses of intravenous gamma globulin (HDIGG). Clin Lab Haematol 1986;8:325-35.
168. Barbui T, Bassan R, Viero P, et al. Pure white cell aplasia treated by high dose intravenous immunoglobulin. Br J Haematol 1984;58:554-5.

169. Breedveld FC, Brand A, van Aken WG. High dose intravenous gamma globulin for Felty's syndrome. J Rheumatol 1985;12: 700-2.

170. Grillot-Courvalin C, Vinci G, Tsapis A, et al. The syndrome of T8 hyperlymphocytosis: Variation in phenotype and cytotoxic activities of granular cells and evaluation of their role in associated neutropenia. Blood 1987;70:1204.

171. Newland AC, Catovsky D, Linch D, et al. Chronic T cell lymphocytosis: A review of 21 cases. Br J Haematol 1984;58:433-42.

172. Loughran TP, Starkebaum G. Large granular lymphocyte leukemia: Report of 38 cases and review of the literature. Medicine 1987;66:397-405.

173. Loughran TP, Coyle T, Sherman MP, et al. Detection of human T-cell leukemia/lymphoma virus, type II, in a patient with large granular lymphocyte leukemia. Blood 1992;80:1116-9.

174. van der Veen JPW, Hack CE, Engelfriet CP, et al. Chronic idiopathic and secondary neutropenia: Clinical and serological investigations. Br J Haematol 1986;63:161-71.

175. Eastlund DT, Charbonneau TT, Steinmetz J. Granulocyte antibody detection to diagnose immune granulocytopenia and transfusion reactions due to leukocyte incompatibility. Hematol Rev 1992; 6:201-13.

176. Rothko K, Kickler TS, Clay ME, et al. Immunoblotting characterization of neutrophil antigenic targets in autoimmune neutropenia. Blood 1989;74:1698-703.

177. Bux J, Robertz-Vaupel GM, Glasmacher A, et al. Autoimmune neutropenia due to NA1 specific antibodies in primary biliary cirrhosis. Br J Haematol 1991;77:121-2.

178. Klaassen RJH, Vlekke ABJ, von dem Borne AEGKr. Neutrophil-bound immunoglobulin in HIV infection is of autoantibody nature. Br J Haematol 1991;77:403-9.

In: Nance ST, ed.
Alloimmunity: 1993 and Beyond
Bethesda, MD: American Association of Blood Banks, 1993

THE EMILY COOLEY MEMORIAL LECTURE

4

Platelet-Specific Alloantigen Systems: History, Clinical Significance and Molecular Biology

Richard H. Aster, MD

RED BLOOD CELL ALLOANTIGENS were identified almost 100 years ago. During the first half of this century, a thorough understanding of red cell alloantigen systems developed at the serologic level, driven by the need to ensure compatibility of transfused red cells and by the discovery that hemolytic disease of the newborn had an alloimmune pathogenesis. Characterization of alloantigen systems expressed on other blood elements such as lymphocytes, granulocytes and platelets began only in the 1950's and 60's when serious consideration was given to using these cells for transfusion purposes and with the recognition that lymphocytes carry alloantigens relevant to organ transplantation. Identification of the first platelet-specific alloantigen system (defined as those normally expressed on platelets but not on red cells or lymphocytes) resulted from studies of two diseases—posttransfusion purpura (PTP) and neonatal alloimmune thrombocytopenic purpura (NATP), both characterized in 1959-62 in the laboratory of Dr. N. R. Shulman at the National Heart, Lung, and Blood Institute. This chapter will review briefly some historical aspects of platelet-specific alloantigen systems, describe the clinical manifestations and pathogenesis of the disorders in which they are involved and summarize the current understanding of their molecular composition and immunogenicity. The chapter will focus

Richard H. Aster, MD, President, The Blood Center of Southeastern Wisconsin and Clinical Professor of Medicine and Pathology, Medical College of Wisconsin, Milwaukee, Wisconsin
(This work was supported, in part, by Grants HL-13629 and HL-44612 from the National Heart, Lung, and Blood Institute.)

on the Pl^{A1} alloantigen, starting with its serologic identification and association with disease and ending with the delineation of its molecular structure about 25 years later. Other platelet alloantigens and systems will be highlighted in the course of discussing this epitope.

Posttransfusion Purpura

Background

The recognition of Pl^{A1} derived from studies of a remarkable complication of blood transfusion: posttransfusion purpura. The first case of PTP described in the literature appears to be that of a woman, reported by Zucker et al in 1959, who developed thrombocytopenia after receiving blood transfusions during cancer therapy.[1] The woman's serum caused agglutination and lysis of normal platelets and inhibited clot retraction. After treatment with corticosteroids, her platelets rose to normal levels in 3 weeks. At about the same time, van Loghem et al encountered a similar patient and found that her serum contained an alloantibody that agglutinated platelets from about 98% of the general population.[2] The alloantigen for which it was specific, designated Zw^a, was shown in family studies to be inherited as a dominant trait. At the National Institutes of Health, we had the good fortune to encounter two patients with similar clinical and serologic findings, enabling us to propose PTP as a distinct clinical entity.[3] One of the patients recovered after 3 weeks of corticosteroid therapy (Fig 4-1). The other improved rapidly after exchange transfusion with whole blood (Fig 4-2). Complement fixation and platelet agglutination showed that antibodies from both patients recognized the same determinant expressed on platelets of 98% of the general population but absent from the patients' own platelets obtained after recovery. Not knowing of van Loghem's studies, we called the alloantigen recognized by these sera Pl^{A1}. An exchange of sera demonstrated that Pl^{A1} was identical to Zw^a.

Pathogenesis

Many cases of PTP have now been described, and the "natural history" of this condition has been well characterized.[4-7] For many years, no satisfactory explanation was advanced to explain how an alloantibody, presumably stimulated by foreign platelets contained in a blood transfusion, could induce the destruction of autologous platelets. Observations made in recent years suggest that several different mechanisms may be operative.

Three groups of investigators have shown that nonsedimentable Pl^{A1} alloantigen accumulates in plasma during the storage of blood in

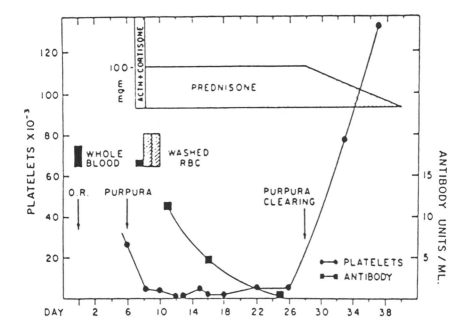

Figure 4-1. Clinical course of a patient alloimmunized against Pl^{A1} who developed posttransfusion purpura following whole blood transfusion. Severe thrombocytopenia and bleeding developed 7 days after transfusion. Anti-Pl^{A1} antibody (measured in arbitrary units) became undetectable just prior to a rise in platelet count at about 27 days. (Used with permission from Shulman et al.[3])

a form capable of binding to Pl^{A1}-negative platelets to provide a target for antibody.[8-10] Shulman directly demonstrated Pl^{A1} in the acute-phase plasma of patients with PTP and performed calculations indicating that these quantities of alloantigen would be sufficient to prime Pl^{A1}-negative platelets for destruction by alloantibody.[10] It is likely that "soluble" Pl^{A1} in stored blood is associated with microparticles shed from platelets,[11,12] although this has not been directly demonstrated. Pl^{A1}-specific alloantibody can be eluted from platelets during the acute stage of the disease.[13,14] Thus, in some patients, PTP may result from the following sequence of events: 1) "soluble" Pl^{A1} alloantigen in transfused blood binds to autologous, Pl^{A1}-negative platelets and, at the same time, triggers the formation of anti-Pl^{A1} alloantibody; 2) antibody binds to Pl^{A1} alloantigen on autologous platelets to promote platelet destruction (Table 4-1). Alternatively, antibody may bind to soluble Pl^{A1} to form immune complexes that bind to platelet Fc receptors. Shulman has suggested that the prolonged course of PTP in some patients (4 weeks or more) reflects the recycling of transfused Pl^{A1} from platelet to platelet.[15]

An alternative explanation for PTP is that platelet-specific *autoantibodies* ("cross-reactive" antibodies) are produced by some patients in paral-

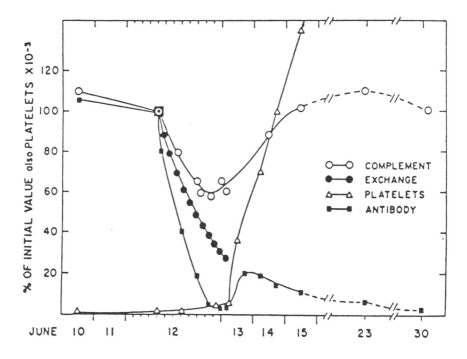

Figure 4-2. Course of a patient alloimmunized against Pl^{A1} who developed posttransfusion purpura and was treated with whole blood exchange transfusion. Thrombocytopenia and bleeding were observed 7 days after blood transfusions were given at the time of open-heart surgery. There was no response to prednisone 50 mg/day, and a 5500 mL whole blood exchange was undertaken over a 16-hour period beginning on day 11. Platelets rose to normal levels over the next 3 days despite a later rebound in antibody levels. (Used with permission from Shulman et al.[3])

lel with anti-Pl^{A1} and that these antibodies are primarily responsible for platelet destruction. Pl^{A1}-specific alloantibodies can be "eluted" from Pl^{A1}-negative platelets following recovery from PTP,[16] but this finding does not confirm autospecificity because substantial amounts of IgG, apparently identical to circulating plasma IgG, are contained in the alpha granules of platelets[17] and should be recovered in eluates prepared under conditions leading to granule disruption. However, an autoimmune pathogenesis is supported by studies in which platelet autoantibodies and severe, transient thrombocytopenia were regularly induced in one species of marmoset injected with platelets from another.[18] At a clinical level, eluates from Pl^{A1}-negative platelets obtained during the acute phase of PTP in several patients were shown to react with both Pl^{A1}-positive and Pl^{A1}-negative target platelets.[13] Berney et al identified an IgM antibody reactive with Pl^{A1}-positive and negative platelets in the recovery plasma from a patient with PTP, but its causal significance was questionable because it was absent from

Table 4-1. Mechanisms Proposed for the Etiology of Posttransfusion Purpura

Passive acquisition of PlA1 antigen	Glycoprotein IIIa carrying PlA1 is present in transfused blood, possibly in the form of microparticles, and binds to recipient platelets. Anti-PlA1 antibody, when formed, recognizes PlA1 on autologous platelets and promotes their destruction.
Immune complexes	PlA1 on transfused glycoprotein IIIa promotes antibody formation and then binds to antibody to produce immune complexes that bind with high affinity to recipient platelets.
Autoantibodies	Platelet-reactive autoantibodies are produced in parallel with the alloimmune response to transfused PlA1, causing destruction of autologous platelets. Eventually, the autoresponse is suppressed, allowing platelets to return to normal.

acute-phase serum.[19] However, Minchinton and coworkers detected an acute-phase IgG antibody in another patient that reacted with autologous platelets as well as PlA1-negative and -positive platelets from normal subjects and disappeared after recovery.[20]

At the Blood Center of Southern Wisconsin, we recently encountered a patient whose clinical course and serologic findings also support the possibility that autoantibodies cause PTP. This individual was a 77-year-old man who received blood transfusions during surgery and developed profound thrombocytopenia and generalized bleeding 13 days later. He recovered in 5 days when treated with prednisone, intravenous gammaglobulin (IVIG) and plasma exchange. His platelets were PlA1-negative. No IgG antibodies were detected, but an IgM antibody specific for the glycoprotein IIb/IIIa complex on autologous platelets and on PlA1-positive and -negative platelets from normal subjects was present. This antibody disappeared after recovery and, unfortunately, lost its activity after being stored frozen for several months. Curiously, this patient never produced demonstrable antibody specific for PlA1.

The proposal that destruction of PlA1-negative platelets in PTP is a consequence of passive absorption of "soluble" PlA1 and/or PlA1-anti-

Pl^{A1} immune complexes by autologous platelets is intriguing, but it is uncertain whether circulating Pl^{A1} antigen could persist for weeks in some patients in the presence of alloantibody. Also questionable is why platelets should be targeted for binding of Pl^{A1} rather than other blood cells that should, in theory, be capable of interacting with platelet microparticles. Patients with PTP often mount a polyspecific immune response against red cells, granulocytes and HLA antigens in addition to producing antibodies against platelet-specific antigens.[21,22] Moreover, transient production of autoantibodies has been demonstrated in association with the alloresponse against erythrocytes.[23-25] Autoantibody production best explains the occasional induction of PTP by leukocyte-reduced red cells[26] and frozen-thawed red blood cells,[27] which are likely to contain enough Pl^{A1} to induce an alloresponse but not to prime autologous Pl^{A1}-negative platelets for destruction.

For these reasons, this author believes that most cases of PTP will eventually be shown to be caused by autoantibodies formed in parallel with alloantibodies reactive with platelet-specific antigens and other alloepitopes. Our finding of a labile IgM autoantibody in acute-phase plasma from a patient with PTP suggests that studies of the reactions of plasma against autologous platelets should be performed as soon as possible after recovery and should include tests for both IgG and IgM.

Clinical and Laboratory Findings

About 90% of the patients who develop PTP are multiparous women receiving a first blood transfusion. Severe thrombocytopenia develops about 5-8 days later accompanied by the production of one or more alloantibodies reactive with platelet-specific alloantigens. Anti-Pl^{A1} is by far the most common. However, antibodies reactive with Pl^{A2} (Zw^b, HPA-1b) and other platelet-specific alloantigens have been described.[28-34] Bleeding is often very severe, and intracranial hemorrhage is a significant risk. It should be kept in mind that acute thrombocytopenia following blood transfusion can be caused by passive infusion of antibodies reactive with the platelet-specific alloantigens.[35-37]

Treatment

Mild cases of posttransfusion purpura without associated bleeding can be managed without specific therapy. Often, however, the platelet count is extremely low and bleeding is life-threatening. Prednisone is routinely administered in large doses, but whether this is beneficial has not been established. Plasmapheresis and exchange transfusion with fresh frozen plasma are often followed by rapid improvement (Fig 4-2) and should be implemented in all patients with life-threatening bleeding. A beneficial effect of IVIG has been described[19,38] and this approach can be considered in addition to or in lieu of plasma exchange. However, the response to plasma exchange may be more rapid. Platelet transfusions are usually ineffective in PTP, and their administration is often followed by severe febrile reactions, sometimes associated with hypotension. Transfusion of Pl^{A1}-negative platelets has been reported to be ineffective[39] and effective,[40] but experience in this area is very limited. For unknown reasons, occasional patients with PTP fail to respond to any of these therapies and have a fatal outcome after many weeks. In one such patient, an apparent response to splenectomy was observed.[41]

Blood transfusions have been administered at a later date to patients recovered from PTP without difficulty in some instances,[42] but recurrences can occur.[15,43] This may be more likely to happen if many years have elapsed between transfusion episodes.[15] It seems reasonable to utilize platelet-depleted products or Pl^{A1}-negative blood when patients with a history of PTP again require transfusion.

Neonatal Alloimmune Thrombocytopenic Purpura

Background

Soon after our recognition of PTP as a clinical entity, four cases were brought to our attention in which infants with severe thrombocytopenia were born to women with normal platelet counts and no history of idiopathic (autoimmune) thrombocytopenic purpura (ITP). Only a few cases of presumptive alloimmune thrombocytopenia had been described up to that time and well-defined alloantibodies reactive with fetal and paternal platelets had not been characterized. When maternal serum from our cases was studied, two were found to contain antibodies specific for Pl^{A1}. Pl^{A1} antigen was detected on platelets of the propositus and the father in these instances.[44] In the other two families, antibodies reactive with an alloantigen carried on platelets from about 50% of the normal population were identified. Initially, this antigen was designated Pl^{B1} on the assumption that it was part of a new platelet-specific alloantigen system. Subsequently, Pl^{B1} was found to be identical with the Class I HLA antigen, HLA-A2.

Pathogenesis

Since our initial report, hundreds of cases of NATP have been described, and it has been found that this condition can be also induced by maternal-fetal transfer of alloantibodies specific for the platelet alloantigens Pl^{A2} (HPA-1b),[45] Ko^a (HPA-2a),[46] Bak^a (HPA-3a),[47,48] Bak^b

(HPA-3b),[49] Pen^a/Yuk^b (HPA-4a),[50] Yuk^a/Pen^b (HPA-4b),[51] Br^a (HPA-5b),[52,53] Br^b (HPA-5a),[54,55] and the low-frequency alloantigens Mo,[56] Tu/Ca[57,58] and Sr^a [59] (Table 4-2). About half of all cases of NATP result from maternal-fetal incompatibility for Pl^{A1}.[60,61] Incompatibility for Br^a/Br^b is the second leading cause.[60] Other alloantigens induce NATP only sporadically in Caucasian populations.

In studies of suspected NATP, platelet-specific alloantibodies are identified only in about half of the cases.[61-63] Presumably, those in which antibodies are not detected are caused by unrecognized platelet-specific alloantigens, are due to antibodies specific for Class I HLA antigens or ABO or have some other etiology, eg, unrecognized infection. When platelet-specific antibodies are absent from maternal serum, high titer, broadly reactive HLA antibodies are more likely to be present[63] and occasional cases of NATP thought to have been caused by alloantibodies reactive with HLA-A2 have been described.[64,65] As noted earlier, two of our original cases of NATP were associated with maternal-fetal incompatibility for HLA-A2.[44] Given the fact that Class I HLA antigens are widely expressed on human tissues with access to the circulation and are found in relatively large quantities soluble in the plasma, it is difficult to envision how HLA-specific alloantibodies could cause isolated neonatal thrombocytopenia. NATP associated with maternal-fetal incompatibility for ABO has been reported,[60] but

Table 4-2. Human Platelet Alloantigen Systems

Alloantigen System	Other Published Names	Allelic Forms	Phenotypic Frequency	Glycoprotein Location
HPA-1	Pl^{A1}, Zw	HPA-1a (Pl^{A1})	72%	GPIIIa
		HPA-1b (Pl^{A2})	26%	Leu$\leftrightarrow$Pro$_{33}$
HPA-2	Ko, Sib	HPA-2a (Ko^b)	85%	GPIb
		HPA-2b (Ko^a)	14%	Thr$\leftrightarrow$Met$_{145}$
HPA-3	Bak, Lek	HPA-3a (Bak^a)	37%	GPIIb
		HPA-3b (Bak^b)	48%	Ile$\leftrightarrow$Ser$_{843}$
HPA-4	Pen, Yuk	HPA-4a (Pen^a)	99%	GPIIIa
		HPA-4b (Pen^b)	<0.1%	Arg$\leftrightarrow$Gin$_{143}$
HPA-5	Br, Hc, Zav	HPA-5a (Br^b)	80%	GPIa
		HPA-5b (Br^a)	19%	
?	Ca, Tu	?	<1%	GPIIIa
?	Mo	?	<1%	GPIIIa
				Pro$\leftrightarrow$Ala$_{407}$
?	Sr^a	?	<1%	GPIIIa

Phenotype frequencies are shown for a Caucasian population only. Significant differences in gene frequencies may be found in Black, Oriental and Native American populations. (Adapted from Newman et al.[109])

a cause-and-effect relationship has been equally difficult to establish because of the widespread tissue distribution of these alloantigens.

Clinical and Laboratory Findings

The natural history of NATP has been described in many reports.[7,15,60,61,66] Its frequency has been estimated at between 1:2000 and 1:5000 births.[67] Mildly affected infants may be asymptomatic. In those with more severe thrombocytopenia, petechial hemorrhages in the skin and mucous membranes are present at birth or appear during the first few hours of life. Megakaryocytes are usually plentiful in the bone marrow, and marrow aspiration is generally not indicated. Occasionally, however, megakaryocytes are markedly decreased or absent.[44,46,64] The maternal platelet count is generally normal, but moderate thrombocytopenia in the mother does not argue against the diagnosis of NATP because the condition sometimes occurs in association with maternal ITP[68] or "gestational" thrombocytopenia, an incidental condition, in itself.[69] As noted, alloantibodies reactive with platelet-specific alloantigens on paternal platelets can be demonstrated in about 50% of cases using a variety of serologic techniques. Occasionally, alloantibodies are undetectable in Pl^{A1}-negative mothers whose offspring are Pl^{A1}-positive. A method for concentrating maternal alloantibodies by absorption and elution with paternal platelets has been described.[70]

In most instances, NATP is a benign, self-limited disorder lasting 2-14 days. However, cases lasting more than 3 months have been described.[48] Reasons for case-to-case variation in the duration of thrombocytopenia are unclear. External or gastrointestinal bleeding, when it occurs, can readily be managed by transfusions. However, intracranial hemorrhage (ICH) occurs prenatally or perinatally in 10-20% of infants with severe thrombocytopenia.

Unfortunately, many cases of ICH associated with NATP occur prenatally.[50,63,71,72] Almost all reported cases of ICH associated with NATP have occurred in association with maternal-fetal incompatibility for Pl^{A1}. The reason for this is uncertain, but the Pl^{A1} alloantigen is known to be expressed on endothelial cells,[73] and it seems possible that damage to endothelium by passively acquired maternal alloantibodies is a contributing factor. Antigens of the Br system are expressed on cultured endothelial cells,[74] but ICH associated with the maternal-fetal incompatibility for Br alloantigens has not been described.

Treatment

Mild, asymptomatic cases often require no specific therapy. Corticosteroids are commonly given, but there is no clear evidence that this is beneficial. Platelets should be transfused to any infant with severe hemorrhage and can help to prevent bleeding in asymptomatic infants. Whenever possible, platelets compatible with the maternal alloantibody should be given. When this is unfeasible, compatible platelets can be obtained from the mother by plateletpheresis (Fig 4-3). Maternal platelets should, of course, be carefully washed to remove alloantibody before being administered. No cases of graft-vs-host disease (GVHD) have been described in association with this treatment, but gamma irradiation is advisable in any transfusion between relatives. Numerous reports of the effectiveness of IVIG in NATP have appeared in recent years,[76-78] and this treatment is worthy of trial. However, IVIG is not always helpful and several days may be required for a response. Exchange transfusion to remove maternal alloantibody is rarely necessary, but can be considered in infants unresponsive to other treatment. There is no role for removal of the spleen in the treatment of NATP.

Since about half of the cases of NATP occur during the first pregnancy,[60,61] it is impossible to anticipate ICH in many instances. As noted, most cases of ICH occur prenatally, sometimes as early as the beginning of the second trimester.[79] In women with a history of NATP who are pregnant again, steps can be taken to minimize the risk of ICH. The presence of a platelet-specific alloantibody during pregnancy is associated with a high probability of moderate-to-severe

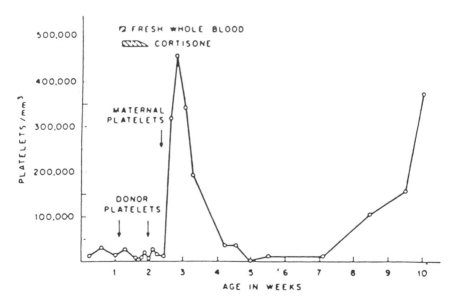

Figure 4-3. Clinical course of an infant with neonatal alloimmune thrombocytopenic purpura (NATP) caused by placental transfer of maternal anti-Pl^{A1}. Random-donor platelets were ineffective, but washed maternal platelets elevated the platelet count to normal. (Used with permission from McIntosh et al.[75])

NATP, but absence of alloantibody does not rule out the possibility of neonatal thrombocytopenia.[80] DNA-based prenatal platelet typing using amniocytes or chorionic villus material is now possible for alloantigens of the Pl^{A1}/Pl^{A2}, Bak^a/Bak^b and Pen^a/Pen^b systems.[81] By this approach, it can be determined with certainty whether the fetus carries the alloantigen for which maternal antibody is specific; testing is indicated whenever the father is heterozygous for the implicated alloantigen.

In infants at risk for NATP, platelet levels can be determined by percutaneous umbilical vein sampling.[82-85] Intrauterine platelet transfusions via the umbilical vein have been given successfully.[86-88] However, this invasive therapy should be reserved for severely affected infants with a high risk of ICH.[85] Prenatal treatment of the mother with IVIG 1 g/kg/week is effective,[83,85,89] and may become the treatment of choice. Whether prenatal corticosteroids are beneficial is uncertain.

Infants at risk for NATP are often delivered by caesarean section, sometimes before term, but whether this reduces the frequency of perinatal ICH is uncertain. It was formerly thought that NATP could be diagnosed early in delivery by sampling scalp blood from the fetus at presentation, but the validity of this approach has recently been questioned.[90]

Molecular Basis of Platelet-Specific Alloantigens

The Pl^A System

In studies done soon after identification of Pl^{A1}, evidence was obtained that the Pl^{A1} epitope is carried on an integral membrane protein.[3] A clue to its specific location was provided by the later finding that the antigen is absent from platelets of patients with Type I Glanzmann's thrombasthenia (GT)[91] known to lack two membrane glycoproteins, designated GPIIb and GPIIIa. It was found that Pl^{A1} coisolates with GPIIIa purified from detergent-solubilized platelets,[92] showing that Pl^{A1} is carried on GPIIIa, rather than GPIIb. The antigen was found to be susceptible to cleavage in situ by trypsin and was totally lost when the GPIIIa molecule was chemically reduced or heated at 100 C. Reactions of anti-Pl^{A1} with its target were unaffected by excess quantities of various sugars, and we concluded that the epitope was determined by a peptide sequence in GPIIIa held in its proper configuration by disulfide bonds. Localization of Pl^{A1} on GPIIIa was later confirmed by others.[93,94]

The next step toward characterizing the Pl^{A1} epitope was made by Newman et al who showed that the Pl^{A1} form of GPIIIa differs slightly from the Pl^{A2} form in its isoelectric point and that the alloepitope is unaffected by the removal of saccharides from GPIIIa by the enzymes

Endo D, Endo O and Endo H.[95] By digestion of GPIIIa with trypsin followed by immunoprecipitation, they localized Pl[A1] to a 17,000 kD fragment of GPIIIa and suggested that the Pl[A1] and Pl[A2] alloepitopes result from subtle amino acid differences in the GPIIIa sequence. Kunicki and coworkers, in quantitative studies of the inheritance of Pl[A1] and GPIIb/IIIa in carriers of the gene for GT, obtained evidence hinting that inheritance of GT and expression of Pl[A1] are controlled by different genes.[96] This suggested that the Pl[A1] epitope might be created by a secondary modification of GPIIIa resulting from intracellular processing. However, these findings can now be explained by the requirement for cosynthesis of GPIIb and GPIIIa for membrane expression of either molecule.[97]

Kornecki et al then showed that Pl[A1] is carried on a 66 kD fragment of GPIIIa produced when intact human platelets are treated with chymotrypsin.[98] Two groups provided evidence that this fragment results from partial digestion of a large disulfide-bonded loop of GPIIIa extending from residues 121 to 348.[99,100] This indicated that the 66 kD fragment consisted of two disulfide-linked chains: a 60 kD fragment extending from residues 349 to 762 and a 17 kD fragment consisting of the 120 N terminal amino acids. The previous studies by Newman in which Pl[A1] was localized to a 17 kD fragment of GPIIIa[95] made the N terminal fragment a candidate to carry Pl[A1], but direct sequencing of a peptide this large posed formidable difficulties. The problem was simplified with the identification of the cDNA sequence of GPIIIa by Fitzgerald and coworkers.[101] We reasoned that, although platelets are anucleate cells, they might contain enough residual mRNA coding for GPIIIa to enable the synthesis of cDNA from an mRNA template.[101] We demonstrated the feasibility of this approach using the polymerase chain reaction to amplify platelet mRNA specific for GPIIIa[102] and, by sequencing the amplification product, showed that the Pl[A1] and Pl[A2] alloantigens are associated with a leucine/proline amino acid polymorphism at position 33 from the N-terminus.[103] Bowditch et al also localized Pl[A1] to this region of GPIIIa by epitope selection of a lambda-gt22 expression library of GPIIIa cDNA fragments.[104] Goldberger and coworkers directly confirmed the relationship between this amino acid substitution and formation of the Pl[A1] and Pl[A2] alloantigens in a heterologous mammalian expression system.[105] The GPIIb/IIIa heterodimer and location of the Pl[A1] epitope are depicted schematically in Fig 4-4.

Despite these advances, the exact location of the epitope recognized by anti-Pl[A1] remains uncertain. Calvette and associates, in an elegant series of studies, deduced the locations of the multiple disulfide linkages in GPIIIa.[107] According to their scheme, the Leu 33/Pro 33 polymorphism associated with Pl[A1] is located in a 13 amino acid loop formed by the linkage of Cys 26 and Cys 38

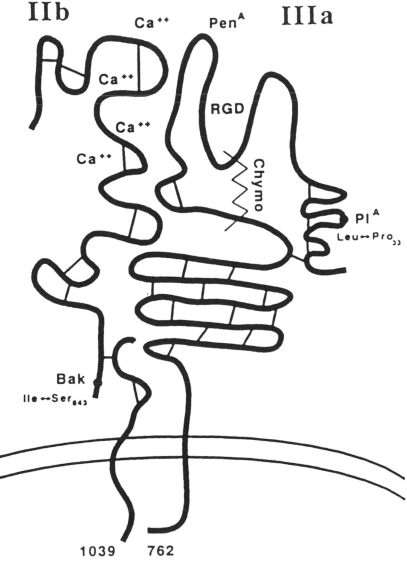

Figure 4-4. Structure of the GPIIb/IIIa heterodimer. The approximate cleavage site for chymo-trypsin and the RGD (arginine-glycine-aspartic acid) binding site in GPIIIa are shown. The PI^A (HPA-1) alloantigens are determined at position 33 from the N terminus of GPIIIa, Bak (HPA-3) alloantigens at position 843 near the C terminus of the GPIIb heavy chain, and Pen/Yuk (HPA-4) by a glycine/arginine substitution at position 143 of GPIIIa, near the RGD binding site. Short-range S-S bonds shown in the disulfide-rich domain of GPIIIa resistant to enzymatic cleavage are schematic and do not represent their actual locations. (Used with permission from Newman.[106])

(Fig 4-5). This region of GPIIIa appears to be linked to a site just proximal to the heavily disulfide-bonded region of GPIIIa by a long-range bond linking Cys 5 to Cys 435. Since chemical reduction of GPIIIa results in loss of the Pl^{A1} epitope,[92] the disulfide bonds presumably stabilize the alloepitope in some way. The possibility exists, therefore, that the epitope is a conformational one, located at a site other than amino acid residue 33. Flug et al found that 13 residue peptides straddling position 33 and corresponding to the Pl^{A1} and Pl^{A2} forms of GPIIIa do not inhibit binding of Pl^{A}-specific alloantibodies to platelets and interpreted this as providing support for this possibility.[108] However, their observation does not prove the point because the failure of anti-Pl^{A1} antibodies to react with reduced GPIIIa[92] already indicated that they were not specific for a linear peptide sequence. Molecular modeling of the 13 amino

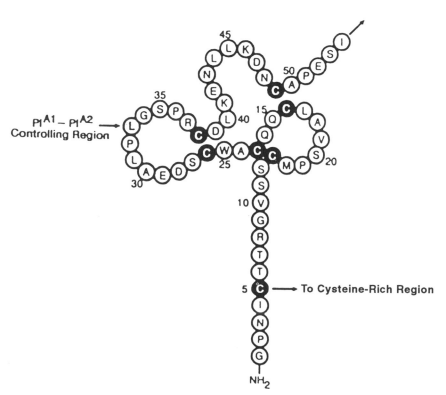

Figure 4-5. Hypothetical model of the secondary structure of the first 54 amino acids of GPIIIa containing seven disulfide-bonded cysteines. The cysteine at residue 5 is coupled to another cysteine at residue 432 in the disulfide-rich region of GPIIIa. (Used with permission from Newman.[106])

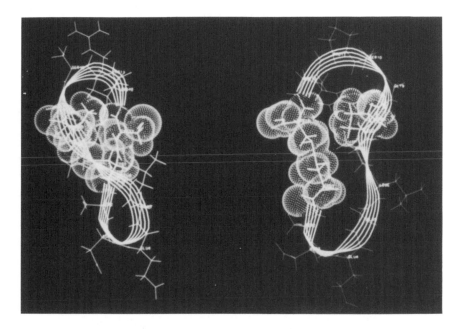

Figure 4-6. Three-dimensional conformation of GPIIIa residues 26-38. Molecular modeling of the loop formed by Cys_{26}-Cys_{38}, performed on an Evans and Sutherland minicomputer using Sybyl energy minimalization software, shows that a proline/leucine substitution at residue 33 causes significant local conformational changes. The loop on the left represents the Leu 33 allele (Pl^{A1}) and the loop on the right represents the Pro 33 (Pl^{A2}) form. The single amino acid substitution causes this small loop to change from a "figure 8" shape (Pl^{A1}) to that of an oblong circle (Pl^{A2}). This difference in conformation appears to facilitate the alloimmune response in posttransfusion purpura and neonatal alloimmune thrombocytopenic purpura. (Used with permission from Newman et al.[109])

acid loops from Cys 26 to Cys 38 shows that the Pl^{A1} (leucine 33) form differs strikingly in its three-dimensional configuration from the Pl^{A2} (proline 33) form (Fig 4-6). Thus, Pl^{A1} and Pl^{A2} should look quite different to Pl^{A}-specific alloantibodies. A distinction between the Pl^{A1} and Pl^{A2} forms of GPIIIa can be made with monoclonal antibodies against the peptide sequence including position 33.[110] However, these antibodies fail to react with GPIIIa in its native form and, therefore, do not recognize the same epitope as human alloantibodies. To date, no synthetic peptide, linear or cyclic, has been shown unequivocally to inhibit anti-Pl^{A1}.

Full characterization of the binding site on GPIIIa for anti-Pl^{A1} is a desirable goal because this information could enable the synthesis of peptides capable of binding anti-Pl^{A1}, which could have therapeutic value. Perhaps monoclonal antibodies with partial specificity for Pl^{A1} on intact GPIIIa will be helpful in this regard.[111-113]

Other Platelet Alloantigen Systems

Currently recognized platelet-specific alloantigens and alloantigen systems and some of their properties are shown in Table 4-2. Several systems have been given more than one designation. Use of a general nomenclature in which systems are designated HPA-1, HPA-2, etc, in the order of their discovery and alleles are designated by the letters a, b, etc,[114] is becoming widely accepted.

Most of the alloantigens identified to date are carried on integrins, a family of heterodimeric protein complexes consisting of alpha and beta chains that mediate cell-to-cell and cell-to-extracellular matrix adhesive interactions.[109] Numerous different alpha and beta subunits have now been cloned and sequenced, and these can combine to form at least 15 different complexes. At least five of these—$\alpha_2\beta_1$, $\alpha_5\beta_1$, $\alpha_6\beta_1$, $\alpha_{IIb}\beta_3$ and $\alpha_v\beta_3$—are expressed on the platelet surface. Integrin α and β subunits are highly conserved in nature, having 18 and 56 cysteine residues respectively in similar locations. Each of the cysteines is disulfide-linked to stabilize the configuration of the mature glycoprotein complex. The amino acid substitutions associated with six of these alloantigen systems and their locations on platelet membrane glycoproteins have now been deduced using PCR-based amplification of platelet mRNA coding for their respective carrier proteins (Table 4-2, Fig 4-7).

The Ko (HPA-2) System

The Ko^a/Ko^b antigens are a diallelic system identified more than 20 years ago with antibodies obtained from transfused patients.[115] Kuijpers and coworkers recently showed that the Ko^a/Ko^b polymorphism is associated with a methionine 145/threonine 145 amino acid polymorphism on platelet glycoprotein Ibα.[116] A closely related polymorphism of GPIbα, designated Sib, has also been described.[117] It was recently learned that the Sib^a alloantigen is associated with a molecular weight polymorphism of GPIb, which is characterized by a difference in the number of 13 amino acid repeat units present in the glycocalicin region of the GPIbα chain.[118] This was unexpected because the four variable 13 amino acid repeats in GPIb that create this molecular polymorphism are about 200 residues away from the Thr 145/Met 145 polymorphism associated with the Ko^a/Ko^b alloantigens. The ability of Sib^a alloantibodies to react only with higher molecular weight forms of GPIb[118] may reflect tight linkage disequilibrium between the high molecular weight forms of GPIbα and the amino acid substitution at position 145 that is essential to the Sib^a epitope. Further studies are required to determine whether the Sib^a and Ko^a epitopes are identical.

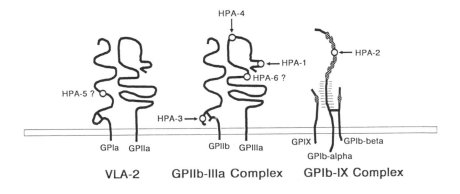

Figure 4-7. Approximate locations of the platelet-specific alloantigens Pl^A (HPA-1), Ko (HPA-2), Bak (HPA-3), Pen/Yuk (HPA-4), Br (HPA-5) and Ca/Tu (HPA-6 ?) on platelet membrane glycoprotein complexes. (Used with permission from Newman et al.[109])

The Bak (Lek, HPA-3) System

An antibody recognizing a platelet-specific alloantigen designated Bak^a was first identified by von dem Borne et al in a case of NATP.[47] Bak^a appears to be identical with Lek^a described by Boizard and Wautier.[119] An antibody recognizing Bak^b, the allele of Bak^a, was found in 1988 by Kickler et al in a patient with PTP.[32] The Bak alloantigen system was shown by immunoblotting to be carried on glycoprotein IIb[120] and is the only reported polymorphism in the heavy chain of the GPIIb/IIIa heterodimeric complex. By an approach similar to that used to characterize the Pl^A system, we found that the Bak^a/Bak^b alloantigen system is associated with an isoleucine 843/serine 843 polymorphism near the C terminus of the GPIIb heavy chain.[121] Take et al found that Bak^a-specific alloantibodies from different individuals vary in their reactions with asialo-GPIIb and suggested that carbohydrate moieties coupled to serine 843 influence the alloimmune response to Bak^a.[122] Goldberger showed that not all anti-Bak antibodies recognize the recombinant precursor form of the GPIIb molecule, Pro-GPIIb, which is not fully glycosylated.[105] Thus, carbohydrate residues added to the GPIIb polypeptide chain during cellular processing may influence the epitope recognized by certain Bak^a-specific alloantibodies. Alloantigens of the Bak system may be similar to the human MN blood group antigens in this respect.[123]

The Pen (Yuk, HPA-4) Alloantigen System

The Pen/Yuk/HPA-4 alloantigen system was independently identified in different laboratories.[50,51] Two groups showed that these alloepitopes are associated with the GPIIIa molecule.[124,125] Utilizing

PCR-based amplification of platelet mRNA coding for GPIIIa, Wang et al [126,127] showed that the Pen[a]/Pen[b] (Yuk[b]/Yuk[a]) polymorphism is associated with an Arg 143/Gln 143 amino acid substitution at residue 143 of GPIIIa. The Pen[b]/Yuk[a] alloantigen is extremely rare in Caucasians but is relatively common among Orientals, and maternal-fetal incompatibility for Pen/Yuk alloantigens is an important cause of NATP among Oriental populations. The Pen/Yuk epitopes lie near the center of a large disulfide-bonded loop of GPIIIa at a site close to the RGD binding domain recognized by the ligands fibrinogen, von Willebrand factor, fibronectin and vitronectin. This appears to explain the ability of anti-Pen/Yuk antibodies to inhibit binding of fibrinogen to platelets[125] and the susceptibility of the Pen/Yuk alloepitope to digestion with chymotrypsin.

The Br (HPA-5) System

The Br[a]/Br[b] alloantigen system was first characterized by Kiefel et al[52,128] and was soon localized by immunochemical studies to glycoprotein Ia, the heavy chain of the GPIa/IIa heterodimeric complex.[129] The same alloantigen system was described independently by Smith et al[130] and Woods and coworkers,[131] who designated it Zav and Hc, respectively. GPIa is the alpha (heavy) chain of the integrin VLA-2 ($\alpha_2\beta_1$) complex, only one or two thousand copies of which are expressed on platelets.[128,129] In contrast, platelets carry about 50,000 copies of the Pl[A] and Bak epitopes. Possibly, this is why NATP associated with Br incompatibility tends to be less severe than that associated with Pl[A], Bak and Pen incompatibility. The amino acid substitution that corresponds to the Br[a]/Br[a] epitopes has recently been determined (Santoso S, Newman P, personal communication).

The Mo Alloantigen

A low frequency (< 0.5%) alloantigen designated Mo was recently identified by Kuijpers et al using serum from a mother who had given birth to a thrombocytopenic infant.[56] By immunochemical studies, Mo was shown to be carried on GPIIIa. By PCR-based amplification and sequencing of cDNA, coding for GPIIIa was linked to a proline 407/alanine 407 amino acid substitution.

The Sr System

A low frequency (< 1%) alloantigen designated Sr[a] carried on GPIIIa was identified by Kroll et al, also using serum from a patient with NATP.[59] Sr[a] resides on a 68 kD proteolytic fragment of GPIIIa and has so far been identified only within the family of the propositus. The amino acid substitution corresponding to the Sr[a] alloepitope has recently been identified (Santoso S, personal communication).

The Ca (Tu) Alloantigen System

In collaboration with a group in Toronto, McFarland et al recently encountered yet another low-incidence alloantigen in studying a case of NATP in which both parents were of Filipino origin.[58] By immunoprecipitation, it was found that the epitope, designated Ca, is carried on glycoprotein IIIa. In an exchange of serum, it was found that Ca is identical with Tu, a low-incidence alloantigen identified by Kekomäki and coworkers in the Finnish population.[57] The Ca/Tu alloantigen has also been localized to a specific amino acid substitution in GPIIIa.[132]

The Gov Alloantigen System

Kelton and coworkers, using serum from transfused patients, recently described an alloantigen system designated Gov[a]/Gov[b], which was shown by immunoprecipitation to be carried on a platelet membrane protein of apparent molecular weight about 175 kD (reduced) and 150 kD (nonreduced).[133] The protein that carries the Gov epitope has not yet been identified, but appears to be distinct from GPIIb/IIIa, GPIb/IX and GPIa/IIa.

The Nak Isoantigen

Ikeda et al described a platelet antigen, Nak[a], using serum from a multitransfused thrombocytopenic patient who was refractory to HLA-matched platelets.[134] Tomiyama et al showed that Nak[a]-specific antibodies react with GPIV (CD36), an 86 kD membrane glycoprotein that may be important for the interaction of platelets with collagen and thrombospondin.[135] Subsequently, it was found that the Nak[a]-negative state is associated with failure to synthesize and express GPIV.[136] Thus, anti-Nak[a] induced by transfusion in persons who are Nak[a]-negative is an isoantibody, rather than an alloantibody. Platelets lacking GPIV appear to function normally.[136]

The Immune Response to Platelet-Specific Alloantigens

Frequency of Alloimmunization

Alloimmunization against the Bak[a]/Pl[A2][137] and Ko[a]/Sib[a][117] alloantigens and the Nak[a] isoantigen[134] was associated with refractoriness to platelet transfusions in several instances. However, fewer than 10% of multitransfused patients and fewer than 1% of multiparous women appear to become sensitized to platelet-specific antigens.[138-140] In a prospective study, it was found that only about 5% of Pl^{A1}-negative women form anti-Pl^{A1} when carrying a Pl^{A1}-positive fetus.[141] Thus, under most circumstances, platelet-specific alloantigens are not highly immunogenic.

The Immune Response to Pl^{A1}

However, a remarkable association between HLA-DR and the formation of Pl^{A1}-specific alloantibodies has been demonstrated. Reznikoff-Etievant found that five of six Pl^{A1}-negative women alloimmunized against Pl^{A1} by pregnancy were positive for the Class I HLA alloantigen HLA-B8 and noted previous examples of this connection from the literature.[142] Two groups subsequently described a strong association between Pl^{A1} alloimmunization and the Class II alloantigen HLA-DR3, which is in close linkage disequilibrium with HLA-B8.[143,144] DeWaal then found an even closer relationship between Pl^{A1} alloimmunization and the Class II alloantigen DRw52 in association with HLA-DR3 or HLA-DRw6.[145] Mueller-Eckhardt et al analyzed HLA phenotypes in 59 Pl^{A1}-negative mothers who had given birth to a Pl^{A1}-positive child but failed to demonstrate a difference in the frequency of DRw52 in responders vs nonresponders and questioned the importance of DRw52 in Pl^{A1} alloimmunization.[146] They also found that DRw6 was even more common in nonresponders than in responders.

Subsequently, DR3 was subdivided into DRw18 and DRw17[147] and DRw52 was split into three subspecificities, DRw52a, b and c[148] by molecular genetic methods. Valentin et al, using restriction fragment length polymorphism analysis, showed that each of 18 Pl^{A1}-negative women alloimmunized against Pl^{A1} had the DRw52a allele at the DR-D3 locus, regardless of their HLA-DRB1 gene product.[149] In contrast, only one of three Pl^{A1}-negative women who gave birth to normal Pl^{A1}-positive children carried the DRw52a gene. The relative risk for immunization against Pl^{A1} in a Pl^{A1}-negative woman positive for DRw52a could not be calculated exactly because none of the alloimmunized women were DRw52 negative; however, it was estimated to be at least 46:1. It was concluded that susceptibility to immunization against Pl^{A1} is very closely linked to DRw52a. Similar observations were made by Decary et al.[150] Together, the studies by Valentin et al[149] and Decary et al[150] found that each of 52 Pl^{A1}-negative "responding" women were positive for HLA-DRw52a. About 30% of "nonresponders" were also HLA-DRw52a-positive, indicating that the DRw52a HLA gene product might be necessary, but is not sufficient to induce alloimmunity against Pl^{A1}.

L'Abbe et al utilized polymerase chain reaction and sequence-specific oligonucleotide probes (PCR-SSOP) to study HLA-DR and HLA-DQ genes in 36 women who formed anti-Pl^{A1} (responders) and 10 who did not (nonresponders) when challenged with the Pl^{A1} alloantigen during pregnancy.[151] They confirmed the close relationship between the gene DRB3*0101 (DRw52a) and responsiveness (odds ratio 24.9). Alloimmunization against Pl^{A1} was even more strongly associated with the gene DQB1*0201 (odds ratio 39.7). This is of particular interest in view of the recognized association of certain DQ phenotypes and autoimmune diseases such as Type I diabetes mellitus, pemphigus vulgaris, rheumatoid arthritis, celiac disease and Sjögren's syndrome.[151] However, the implicated genes were also present in some nonresponders. Sequencing studies showed that the failure of nonresponders to form antibody could not be explained by variant forms of the implicated genes. It was suggested that nonresponders may be able to present Pl^{A1} antigen to T cells but differ from responders in some other aspect of the immune response, eg, in their T-cell repertoire.

Yassai and coworkers analyzed HLA phenotypes in 20 additional Pl^{A1}-negative subjects who were immunized against Pl^{A1} and, combining their data with those reported by others, estimated the relative risk of alloimmunization in Pl^{A1}-negative subjects positive for DR52a to be 141:1.[152] However two of the 20 individuals they studied were positive for DR52b, rather than DR52a. Thus, Pl^{A1} alloimmunization can occur in association with HLA-DR52a, 52b and 52c. The same group of workers used one-way PCR to study V, J and D gene utilization in T-cell receptor beta chains of their patients and observed preferential utilization of the genes VB4.1, VB19.1 and VB9.1 in one alloimmunized subject.[152] They then applied an innovative strategy ("spectratyping") to evaluate the immune response of susceptible individuals to Pl^{A1} in vitro. In these studies, T cells were obtained from immunized women at the time they gave birth to a Pl^{A1}-positive infant and at 6 and 18 months after the birth. The CDR3 region of the T-cell beta chain mRNA was then amplified using a primer specific for the C (or J) region specific for each of the family of V genes. Primers were chosen so that the amplification products were relatively short (about 200 bp) so that they could be resolved on a denaturing polyacrylamide gel. The resulting "spectratypes" provide a measure of CDR3 region composition within each of the V gene "families." Within V gene families, significant differences were observed in CDR3 composition at the three different time intervals. In-vitro studies were then performed in which T cells from an alloimmunized patient were stimulated by sonicated platelet membranes in the presence and absence of T-cell growth factor and the CDR3 regions within the VB3 and VB4 families were studied by "spectratyping." Sonicated platelet membranes, but not a tridecapeptide corresponding to amino acid residues 27-39 of GPIIIa, produced significant T-cell stimulation and unique CDR3 patterns (Fig 4-8).

The Immune Response to Br^a

Mueller-Eckhardt et al performed HLA phenotyping on 16 individuals immunized against the Br^a antigen carried on glycoprotein Ia[153] and found a strong association between the alloresponse to this determinant and the presence of HLA-DRw6, which is closely linked to DRw52a.

The Immune Response to Pl^{A2}

Kuijpers et al utilized serologic and cellular typing to determine the phenotypes of 10 women homozygous for Pl^{A1} who formed antibodies against the Pl^{A2} alloantigen.[154] Five of the 10 responders were positive for HLA-DRw52a and no statistically significant association between response to Pl^{A2} and DR phenotype was observed. From population studies, the authors estimated that the Pl^{A1} alloantigen was about 1000 times more immunogenic than Pl^{A2}. It was suggested that the Pl^{A2} form of GPIIIa (GPIIIa-proline 33) is perhaps not capable of being presented by any DR molecule and that an association might be found between

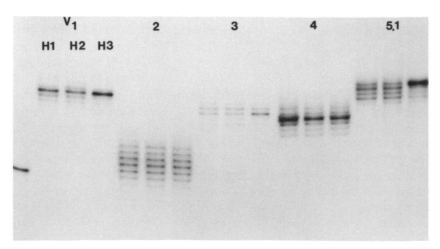

Figure 4-8. "Spectratype" analysis of peripheral blood mononuclear cells obtained from a woman alloimmunized against Pl^{A1}. Samples H1, H2 and H3 were obtained at the time of delivery of a Pl^{A1}-positive infant and 6 and 18 months later, respectively. Results are shown for members of the VB gene families 1-5 coding for the CDR region of the T-cell receptor beta chain. A progressive change in VB4 and VB5.1 and relative stability of the VB 1-3 patterns are apparent. (Used with permission from Yassai et al.[152])

Pl^{A2} sensitization and DQ or DP gene products. The authors interpreted their data to imply that an oligopeptide from the Pl^{A1} form of GPIIIa is presented much more efficiently by HLA-DRw52a than the comparable oligopeptide from the Pl^{A2} form, ie, the immune response is dramatically affected by a single amino acid substitution.

Future Prospects

The association between HLA-DR and susceptibility to alloimmunization against Pl^{A1} is closer than that of any other known alloimmune response. It seems possible that the further studies of the molecular basis for Pl^{A1} alloimmunization may provide the first complete understanding of the alloresponse to a clinically significant antigen.

Acknowledgments

I wish to express my gratitude to the many coworkers at The Blood Center of Southeastern Wisconsin who have collaborated with me in research over a period of many years, especially Drs. Gary Becker, Douglas Christie, Philip Cimo, Rene Duquesnoy, Donald Filip, Jerome Gottschall, Kyou Sup Han, Thomas Kunicki, Janice McFarland, Jay Menitove, Diego Mezzano, Robert Montgomery, Betsy Neahring, Peter Newman, Jaime Pereira, Glenn Rodey, Nancy Szatkowski, Peter Tomasulo, Gian Visentin, Hans Wadenvik, Lee Ann Weitekamp and Guo-Guant Wu. The outstanding technical support provided by Janice Collins, Brian Curtis, Sheila Ford, Mitch Gajewski, Lanette Kagen, Steven Letellier, Bonnie Miskovich, Kurt Wolfmeyer and many others is gratefully acknowledged. I am indebted to the National Heart, Lung, and Blood Institute for its support of my research program over the past 25 years. Finally, I would like to express my gratitude to my mentors in research, Drs. William Beierwaltes, N. R. Shulman and James Jandl.

References

1. Zucker MB, Ley AB, Borrelli J, et al. Thrombocytopenia with a circulating platelet agglutinin, platelet lysin and clot retraction inhibitor. Blood 1959;14:148-61.
2. van Loghem JJ Jr, Dorfmeijer H, van der Hart M. Serological and genetical studies on a platelet antigen (Zw). Vox Sang 1959; 4:161-9.
3. Shulman NR, Aster RH, Leitner A, Hiller MC. Immunoreactions involving platelets. V. Post-transfusion purpura due to a com-

plement-fixing antibody against a genetically controlled platelet antigen. A proposed mechanism for thrombocytopenia and its relevance in "autoimmunity." J Clin Invest 1961;40:1597-620.

4. Mueller-Eckhardt C. Post-transfusion purpura. Br J Haematol 1986;64:419-24.

5. Vogelsang G, Kickler TS, Bell WR. Post-transfusion purpura: A report of five patients and a review of the pathogenesis and management. Am J Hematol 1986;21:259-67.

6. Waters AH. Post-transfusion purpura. Blood Rev 1989;3:83-7.

7. Aster RH, George JN. Thrombocytopenia due to enhanced platelet destruction by immunologic mechanisms. In: Williams WJ, Beutler E, Erslev AJ, Lichtman LA, eds. Hematology. 4th ed. New York, NY: McGraw-Hill, 1990:1370-97.

8. Kickler TS, Ness PM, Herman JH, Bell WR. Studies on the pathophysiology of posttransfusion purpura. Blood 1986;68: 347-50.

9. Dieleman LA, Brand A, Claas FHJ, et al. Acquired Zw^a antigen on Zw^a negative platelets demonstrated by Western blotting. Br J Haematol 1989;72:539-42.

10. Shulman NR. Posttransfusion purpura: Clinical features and the mechanism of platelet destruction. In: Nance SJ, ed. Clinical and basic science aspects of immunohematology. Arlington, VA: American Association of Blood Banks, 1991:137-54.

11. George JN, Pickett EB, Heinz R. Platelet membrane microparticles in blood bank fresh frozen plasma and cryoprecipitate. Blood 1986;68:307-9.

12. Abrams CS, Ellison N, Budzynski AZ, Shattil SJ. Direct detection of activated platelets and platelet-derived microparticles in humans. Blood 1990;75:128-38.

13. Pegels JG, Bruynes ECE, Engelfriet CP, von dem Borne AEGKr. Post-transfusion purpura: A serological and immunochemical study. Br J Haematol 1981;49:521-30.

14. von dem Borne AEGKr, van der Plas-van Dalen CM. Further observation on post-transfusion purpura (PTP) (letter). Br J Haematol 1985;61:374-5.

15. Shulman NR, Jordan JV. Platelet immunology. In: Colman RW, Harsch J, Marder VJ, Salzman EW, eds. Hemostasis and thrombosis. Philadelphia, PA: J. B. Lippincott, 1987:452-529.

16. Taaning E, Skov F. Elution of anti-Zw^a (-Pl^{A1}) from autologous platelets after normalization of platelet count in post-transfusion purpura. Vox Sang 1991;60:40-4.

17. George JN. Platelet IgG: Measurement, interpretation, and clinical significance. Prog Hemost Thromb 1991;10:97-126.

18. Barnhart DD, Gengozian N. Actively induced thrombocytopenia in the marmoset. A possible autoimmune model. Clin Exp Immunol 1975;21:493-500.

19. Berney SI, Metcalfe P, Wathen NC, Waters AH. Post-transfusion purpura responding to a high dose intravenous IgG: Further observations on pathogenesis. Br J Haematol 1985;61:627-32.
20. Minchinton RM, Cunningham I, Cole-Sinclair M, et al. Autoreactive platelet antibody in post-transfusion purpura. Aust NZ J Med 1990;20:111-15.
21. Slichter SJ. Post-transfusion purpura: Response to steroids and association with red blood cell and lymphocytotoxic antibodies. Br J Haematol 1982;50:599-605.
22. Puig N, Sayas MJ, Montoro JA, et al. Post-transfusion purpura as the main manifestation of a trilineal transfusion reaction, responsive to steroids: Flow-cytometric investigation of granulocyte and platelet antibodies. Ann Hematol 1991;62:232-4.
23. Polesky HF, Bove JR. A fatal hemolytic transfusion reaction with autologous autohemolysis. Transfusion 1964;4:285-92.
24. Alpaugh K, Sysko-Stein L, Lusch C, et al. Autoanti-Jk^a associated with hemolysis after transfusion with Jk(a+) red cells. Lab Med 1989;20:682-4.
25. Shirey RS, Ness PM. New concepts of delayed hemolytic transfusion reactions. In: Nance SJ, ed. Clinical and basic science aspects of immunohematology. Arlington, VA: American Association of Blood Banks, 1991:179-97.
26. Kalish RI, Jacobs B. Post-transfusion purpura: Initiation by leukocyte-poor red cells in a polytransfused woman. Vox Sang 1987;53:169-72.
27. Godeau B, Fromont P, Bettaieb A, et al. Relapse of posttransfusion purpura after transfusion with frozen-thawed red cells. Transfusion 1991;31:189-90.
28. Taaning E, Morling N, Ovesen H, Svejgaard A. Post-transfusion purpura and anti-Zw^b(-Pl^{A2}). Tissue Antigens 1985;26:143-6.
29. Keimowitz RM, Collins J, Davis K, Aster RH. Post-transfusion purpura associated with alloimmunization against the platelet-specific antigen, Bak^a. Am J Hematol 1986;21:79-88.
30. Simon TL, Collins J, Kunicki TJ, et al. Posttransfusion purpura associated with alloantibody specific for the platelet for the platelet antigen, Pen^a. Am J Hematol 1988;29:38-40.
31. Chapman JF, Murphy MF, Berney SI, et al. Post-transfusion purpura associated with anti-Bak^a and anti-Pl^{A2} platelet antibodies and delayed haemolytic transfusion reaction. Vox Sang 1987;52:313-17.
32. Kickler TS, Herman JH, Furihata K, et al. Identification of Bak^b, a new platelet-specific antigen associated with posttransfusion purpura. Blood 1988;71:894-8.
33. Kiefel V, Santoso S, Glöckner WM, et al. Posttransfusion purpura associated with an anti-Bak^b. Vox Sang 1989;56:93-7.

34. Christie DJ, Pulkrabek S, Putnam JL, et al. Posttransfusion purpura due to an alloantibody reactive with glycoprotein Ia/IIa (anti-HPA-5b). Blood 1991;77:2785-9.
35. Ballem PJ, Buskard NA, Decary F, Doubroff P. Post-transfusion purpura secondary to passive transfer of anti-Pl^{A1} by blood transfusion. Br J Haematol 1987;66:113-4.
36. Scott EP, Moiland-Bergeland J, Dalmasso AP. Posttransfusion thrombocytopenia associated with passive transfusion of a platelet-specific antibody. Transfusion 1988;28:73-6.
37. Warkentin ET, Smith JW, Hayward CPM, et al. Thrombocytopenia caused by passive transfusion of anti-glycoprotein Ia/IIa alloantibody (anti-HPA-5b). Blood 1992;79:2480-4.
38. Mueller-Eckhardt C, Kiefel V. High-dose IgG for post-transfusion purpura—revisited. Blut 1988;57:163-7.
39. Gerstner JB, Smith MJ, Davis KD, et al. Post-transfusion purpura: Therapeutic failure of Pl^{A1}-negative platelet transfusion. Am J Hematol 1979;6:71-5.
40. Brecher ME, Moore SB, Letendre L. Post-transfusion purpura: The therapeutic value of Pl^{A1}-negative platelets. Transfusion 1990;30:433-5.
41. Cunningham CC, Lind SE. Apparent response of refractory post-transfusion purpura to splenectomy. Am J Hematol 1989;30:112-3.
42. Lau P, Sholtis CM, Aster RH. Post-transfusion purpura: An enigma of alloimmunization. Am J Hematol 1980;9:331-6.
43. Budd JL, Wiegers SE, O'Hara JM. Relapsing post-transfusion purpura. A preventable disease. Am J Med 1985;78:361-6.
44. Shulman NR, Aster RH, Pearson HA, Hiller MC. Immunoreactions involving platelets. VI. Reactions of maternal isoantibodies responsible for neonatal purpura. Differentiation of a second platelet antigen system. J Clin Invest 1962;41:1059-69.
45. Mueller-Eckhardt C, Becker T, Weisheit M, et al. Neonatal alloimmune thrombocytopenia due to feto-maternal Zw^b incompatibility. Vox Sang 1986;50:94.
46. Bizzaro N, Dianese G. Neonatal alloimmune amegakaryocytosis (case report). Vox Sang 1988;54:112-4.
47. von dem Borne AEGKr, von Riesz E, Verheugt FW, et al. Bak^a, a new platelet-specific antigen involved in neonatal allo-immune thrombocytopenia. Vox Sang 1980;39:113-20.
48. Miller DT, Etzel RA, McFarland JG, et al. Prolonged neonatal alloimmune thrombocytopenic purpura associated with anti-Bak(a). Two cases in siblings. Am J Perinatol 1987;4:55-8.
49. McGrath K, Minchinton R, Cunningham I, Ayberk H. Platelet anti-Bak^b antibody associated with neonatal alloimmune thrombocytopenia. Vox Sang 1989;57:182-4.

50. Friedman JM, Aster RH. Neonatal alloimmune thrombocytopenic purpura and congenital porencephaly in two siblings associated with a "new" maternal antiplatelet antibody. Blood 1985; 65:1412-5.
51. Shibata Y, Matsuda I, Miyaji T, Ichikawa Y. Yuk^a, a new platelet antigen involved in two cases of neonatal alloimmune thrombocytopenia. Vox Sang 1986;50:177-80.
52. Kiefel V, Santoso S, Katzmann B, Mueller-Eckhardt C. A new platelet-specific alloantigen Br^a. Report of four cases with neonatal alloimmune thrombocytopenia. Vox Sang 1988;54:101-6.
53. Kaplan C, Morel-Kopp MC, Kroll H, et al. HPA-5b (Br^a) neonatal alloimmune thrombocytopenia: Clinical and immunological analysis of 39 cases. Br J Haematol 1991;78:425-9.
54. Betaieb A, Fromont P, Rodet M, et al. Br^b: A platelet alloantigen involved in neonatal alloimmune thrombocytopenia. Vox Sang 1991;60:230-4.
55. Kiefel V, Schechter Y, Atlas D, et al. Neonatal alloimmune thrombocytopenia due to anti-Br^b (HPA-5a). Vox Sang 1991;60: 244-5.
56. Kuijpers RWAM, Simsek S, Faber NM, et al. Single point mutation in human glycoprotein IIIa is associated with a new platelet-specific alloantigen (Mo) involved in neonatal alloimmune thrombocytopenia. Blood 1993;81:70-6.
57. Kekomäki R, Jouhikainen T, Ollikainen J, et al. A new platelet alloantigen, Tu^a, on glycoprotein IIIa associated with neonatal alloimmune thrombocytopenia in two families. Br J Haematol 1993;83:306-10.
58. McFarland JG, Blanchette VE, Collins J, et al. Neonatal alloimmune thrombocytopenia due to a new platelet-specific alloantibody. Blood 1993 (in press).
59. Kroll H, Kiefel V, Santoso S, Mueller-Eckhardt C. Sr^a, a private platelet antigen on glycoprotein IIIa associated with neonatal alloimmune thrombocytopenia. Blood 1990;76:2296-302.
60. Mueller-Eckhardt C, Kiefel V, Grubert A, et al. 348 cases of suspected neonatal alloimmune thrombocytopenia. Lancet 1989;1:363-6.
61. Aster RH, McFarland JG. Neonatal alloimmune thrombocytopenic purpura. In: Bern MM, Frigoletto N, eds. Hematologic contributions to fetal health. New York, NY: Alan R. Liss,1990: 349-60.
62. Kunicki TJ, Aster RH. Qualitative and quantitative test for platelet alloantibodies and drug-dependent antibodies. In: McMillan R, ed. Immune cytopenias. New York, NY: Churchill-Livingstone. 1983:49-67.
63. Aster RH. Clinical significance of platelet-specific antigens and antibodies. In: Advances in immunobiology. Blood cell antigens

and bone marrow transplantation. New York, NY: Alan R. Liss, 1984:103-18.

64. Evans DIK. Immune amegakaryocytic thrombocytopenia of the newborn: Association with anti-HLA-A2. J Clin Pathol 1987;40:258.

65. Chow MP, Sun KJ, Yung CH, et al. Neonatal alloimmune thrombocytopenia due to HLA-A2 antibody. Acta Haematol 1992;87:153-5.

66. Andrew M, Barr RD. Increased platelet destruction in infancy and childhood. Semin Thromb Hemost 1982;8:248-62.

67. Blanchette V. Neonatal alloimmune thrombocytopenia: A clinical perspective. Curr Stud Hematol Blood Transfus 1988;54:112-26.

68. van Leeuwen EF, von dem Borne AEGKr, Oudesluijs-Murphy AM, Ras-Zeijlmans GJM. Neonatal alloimmune thrombocytopenia complicated by maternal autoimmune thrombocytopenia. Br Med J 1980;281:27.

69. Burrows RF, Kelton JG. Alloimmune neonatal thrombocytopenia associated with incidental maternal thrombocytopenia. Am J Hematol 1990;35:43-4.

70. Mueller-Eckhardt C, Kayser W, Forster C, et al. Improved assay for detection of platelet-specific Pl^{A1} antibodies in neonatal alloimmune thrombocytopenia. Vox Sang 1982;43:76-81.

71. Burrows RF, Caco CC, Kelton JG. Neonatal alloimmune thrombocytopenia: Spontaneous in utero intracranial hemorrhage. Am J Hematol 1988;28:98-102.

72. Manson J, Speed I, Abbott K, Crompton J. Congenital blindness porencephaly and neonatal thrombocytopenia: A report of four cases. J Child Neurol 1988;3:120-4.

73. Leeksma OC, Giltay JL, Zandbergen-Spaargaren J, et al. The platelet alloantigen Zw^{a} or Pl^{A1} is expressed by cultured endothelial cells. Br J Haematol 1987;66:369-73.

74. Giltay JC, Brinkman H-JM, Vlekke A, et al. The platelet glycoprotein Ia-IIa-associated Br-alloantigen system is expressed by cultured endothelial cells. Br J Haematol 1990;75:557-60.

75. McIntosh S, O'Brien RT, Schwartz AD, Pearson HA. Neonatal isoimmune purpura: Response to platelet infusions. J Pediatr 1973;82:1020-7.

76. Derycke M, Dreyfus M, Ropert JC, Tchernia G. Intravenous immunoglobulin for neonatal isoimmune thrombocytopenia. Arch Dis Child 1985;60:667.

77. Beck R, Reid DM, Lazarte R. Intravenous gamma globulin therapy for neonatal alloimmune thrombocytopenia. Am J Perinatol 1988;5:79-82.

78. Mueller-Eckhardt C, Kiefel V, Grubert A. High-dose IgG treatment for neonatal alloimmune thrombocytopenia. Blut 1989; 59:145-6.

79. Giovangrandi Y, Daffos C, Kaplan C, et al. Very early intracranial haemorrhage in alloimmune fetal thrombocytopenia. Lancet 1990;2:310.
80. McFarland JG, Frenzke M, Aster RH. Testing of maternal sera in pregnancies at risk for neonatal alloimmune thrombocytopenia. Transfusion 1989;29:128-33.
81. McFarland JG, Aster RH, Bussel JB, et al. Prenatal diagnosis of neonatal alloimmune thrombocytopenia using allele-specific oligonucleotide probes. Blood 1991;78:2276-82.
82. Lynche L, Bussel J, Goldberg JD, et al. The in utero diagnosis and management of alloimmune thrombocytopenia. Prenat Diagn 1988;8:329-31.
83. Bussel JB, Berkowitz RL, McFarland JG, et al. Antenatal treatment of neonatal alloimmune thrombocytopenia. N Engl J Med 1988;319:1374-8.
84. Scioscia AL, Grannum PAT, Copel JA, Hobbins JC. The use of percutaneous umbilical blood sampling in immune thrombocytopenic purpura. Am J Obstet Gynecol 1988;159:1066-8.
85. Bussel J, Kaplan C, McFarland JG. Recommendations for the evaluation and treatment of neonatal autoimmune and alloimmune thrombocytopenia. Thromb Haemost 1991;65:631-4.
86. Kaplan C, Daffos F, Forestier F, et al. Management of alloimmune thrombocytopenia: Antenatal diagnosis and in utero transfusion of maternal platelets. Blood 1988;72:340-3.
87. Nicolini U, Rodeck CH, Kochenour NK, et al. In utero platelet transfusion for alloimmune thrombocytopenia. Lancet 1988; 2:506.
88. Murphy MF, Pullon HWH, Metcalfe P, et al. Management of fetal alloimmune thrombocytopenia by weekly in utero platelet transfusions. Vox Sang 1990;58:45-9.
89. Levine AB, Berkowitz RL. Neonatal alloimmune thrombocytopenia. Semin Perinatol 1991;15(Suppl 2):35-40.
90. Christiaens GCML, Helmerhorst FM. Validity of intrapartum diagnosis of fetal thrombocytopenia. Am J Obstet Gynecol 1987;157:864-5.
91. Kunicki TJ, Aster RH. Deletion of the platelet-specific alloantigen Pl^{A1} from platelets in Glanzmann's thrombasthenia. J Clin Invest 1978;61:1225.
92. Kunicki TJ, Aster RH. Isolation and immunologic characterization of the human platelet alloantigen, Pl^{A1}. Mol Immunol 1979; 16:353-60.
93. Lane J, Brown M, Bernstein I, et al. Serological and biochemical analysis of the Pl^{A1} alloantigen of human platelets. Br J Haematol 1982;50:351-9.

94. McMillan R, Mason D, Tani P, Schmidt GM. Evaluation of platelet surface antigens: Localization of the Pl^{A1} alloantigen. Br J Haematol 1982;51:297-304.

95. Newman PJ, Martin LS, Knipp NA, Kahn RA. Studies on the nature of the human platelet alloantigen, Pl^{A1}. Localization to a 17,000-dalton polypeptide. Mol Immunol 1985;22:719-29.

96. Kunicki TJ, Pidard D, Cazenave JP, et al. Inheritance of the human platelet alloantigen, Pl^{A1}, in Type I Glanzmann's thrombasthenia. J Clin Invest 1981;67:717-24.

97. Rosa JP, McEver RP. Processing and assembly of the integrin, glycoprotein IIb-IIIa in HEL cells. J Biol Chem 1989;264:12596-603.

98. Kornecki E, Chung S-Y, Holt JC, et al. Identification of Pl^{A1} alloantigen domain on a 66 kDa protein derived from glycoprotein IIIa of human platelets. Biochim Biophys 1985;818:285-90.

99. Niewiarowski S, Norton KJ, Eckardt A, et al. Structural and functional characterization of major platelet membrane components derived by limited proteolysis of glycoprotein IIIa. Biochem Biophys Acta 1989;983:91-9.

100. Beer J, Coller BS. Evidence that platelet glycoprotein IIIa has a large disulfide-bonded loop that is susceptible to proteolytic cleavage. J Biol Chem 1989;263:17564-73.

101. Fitzgerald LA, Steiner B, Rall SC, et al. Protein sequence of endothelial glycoprotein IIIa derived from a cDNA clone. Identity with platelet glycoprotein IIIa and similarity to "integrin." J Biol Chem 1987;262:3936-9.

102. Newman PJ, Gorski J, White GC, et al. Enzymatic amplification of platelet-specific mRNA using the polymerase chain reaction. J Clin Invest 1988;82:739-43.

103. Newman PJ, Derbes R, Aster RH. The human platelet alloantigens, Pl^{A1} and Pl^{A2}, are associated with a leucine 33/proline 33 amino acid polymorphism in membrane glycoprotein IIIa and are distinguishable by DNA typing. J Clin Invest 1989;83:1778-82.

104. Bowditch RD, Tani PH, Halloran CE, et al. Localization of a Pl^{A1} epitope to the amino-terminal 66 residues of platelet glycoprotein IIIa. Blood 1992;79:559-62.

105. Goldberger A, Kolodziej M, Poncz M, et al. Effect of single amino acid substitutions on the formation of the Pl^{A} and Bak alloantigenic epitopes. Blood 1991;78:681-7.

106. Newman PJ. Platelet GPIIb-IIIa: Molecular variations and alloantigens. Thromb Haemost 1991;666:111-8.

107. Calvete JJ, Henchen A, Gonzalez-Rodriquez J. Assignment of disulphide bonds in human platelet GPIIIa. A disulphide pattern for the beta-subunits of the integrin family. Biochem J 1991;273:63-71.

108. Flug F, Espinola R, Liu LX, et al. A 13-mer peptide straddling the leucine 33/proline 33 polymorphism in glycoprotein IIIa does not define the Pl^{A1} epitope. Blood 1991;77:1964-9.
109. Newman PJ, McFarland JG, Aster RH. The alloimmune thrombocytopenias. In: Loscalzo J, Schafer AI, eds. Thrombosis and hemorrhage. Cambridge, MA: Blackwell Scientific 1993 (in press).
110. Ryckewaert JJ, Schweizer B, Chapel A, Marguerie G. Production of anti-Pl^{A1} monoclonal antibodies. J Lab Clin Med 1992;119:52-6.
111. Santoso S, Lohmeyer J, Rennich H, et al. Platelet surface antigens: Analysis by monoclonal antibodies. I. Immunological and biochemical studies. Blut 1984;48:161-70.
112. Xi X, Zhao Y, Jiang H, et al. Competitive binding of a monoclonal antibody SZ-21 with anti-Pl^{A1} antibodies and its potential for clinical application. Nouv Rev Fr Hematol 1992;34:239-42.
113. Lin-Xing L, Nardi M, Flug F, Karpatkin S. Development of a monoclonal antibody capable of differentiating platelet Pl^{A1}/Pl^{A1}, Pl^{A1}/Pl^{A2}, and Pl^{A2}/Pl^{A2} genotypes. Br J Haematol 1992;81:113-7.
114. von dem Borne AEGKr, Decary F. Nomenclature of platelet-specific antigens. Hum Immunol 1990;29:1-2.
115. Marcelli-Barge A, Poirier JC, Dausset J. Allo-antigens and allo-antibodies of the Ko system, serological and genetic study. Vox Sang 1973;24:1-11.
116. Kuijpers RWAM, Faber NN, Cuypers HTM, von dem Borne AEGKr. The N-terminal globular domain of human glycoprotein Ibα has a methionine 145/threonine 145 amino acid polymorphism which is associated with the HPA-2 (Ko) alloantigens. J Clin Invest 1993. (in press).
117. Saji H, Maruya E, Fujii H, et al. New platelet antigen, Sib^a, involved in platelet transfusion refractoriness in a Japanese man. Vox Sang 1989;56:283-7.
118. Ishida Y, Saji H, Maruya E, Furihata K. Human platelet-specific antigen, Sib^a, is associated with the molecular weight polymorphism of glycoprotein Ib-alpha. Blood 1991;78:1722-9.
119. Boizard B, Wautier JL. Lek^a, a new platelet antigen absent in Glanzmann's thrombasthenia. Vox Sang 1984;46:47-54.
120. van der Schoot CE, Wester M, von dem Borne AEGKr, Huisman HG. Characterization of platelet-specific alloantigens by immunoblotting: Localization of Zw and Bak antigens. Br J Haematol 1986;64:715-23.
121. Lyman S, Aster RH, Visentin GP, Newman PJ. Polymorphism of human platelet membrane glycoprotein IIb associated with a Bak^a/Bak^b alloantigen system. Blood 1990;75:2343-8.
122. Take H, Tomiyama Y, Shibata Y, et al. Demonstration of the heterogeneity of epitopes of the platelet-specific alloantigen, Bak^a. Br J Haematol 1990;76:395-400.

123. Sadler JE, Paulson JC, Hill RL. The role of sialic acid in the expression of human MN blood group antigens. J Biol Chem 1979;254:2112-9.

124. Shibata Y, Morri H. A new platelet-specific alloantigen system, Yuk^a/Yuk^b, is located on platelet membrane glycoprotein IIIa. Proc Japan Acad 1987;63:36-8.

125. Furihata K, Nugent DJ, Bissonette A, et al. On the association of the platelet-specific alloantigen Pen^a with glycoprotein IIIa. Evidence for heterogeneity of glycoprotein IIIa. J Clin Invest 1987;80:1624-30.

126. Wang R, Furihata K, McFarland JG, et al. An amino acid polymorphism within the RGD binding domain of platelet membrane glycoprotein IIIa is responsible for the formation of the Pen^a/Pen^b alloantigen system. J Clin Invest 1992;90:2038-43.

127. Wang L, Juji T, Shibata Y, et al. Sequence variation of human platelet membrane glycoprotein IIIa associated with the Yuk^a/Yuk^b alloantigen system. Proc Japan Acad 1991;67:102-6.

128. Kiefel V, Santoso S, Katzmann B, Mueller-Eckhardt C. The Br^a/Br^b alloantigen system on human platelets. Blood 1989;73:2219-23.

129. Santoso S, Kiefel V, Mueller-Eckhardt C. Immunochemical characterization of the new platelet alloantigen system, Br^a/Br^b. Br J Haematol 1989;72:191-8.

130. Smith JW, Kelton JG, Horsewood P, et al. Platelet-specific alloantigens on the platelet glycoprotein Ia/IIa complex. Br J Haematol 1989;72:534-8.

131. Woods VL Jr, Pischel KD, Avery ED, Bluestein HG. Antigenic polymorphism of human very late activation protein-2 (platelet glycoprotein Ia-IIa). Platelet alloantigen Hc^a. J Clin Invest 1989; 83:978-85.

132. Wang R, McFarland JG, Kekomäki R, Newman PJ. Amino acid 489 is encoded by a mutational "hot spot" on the β3 integrin chain: The Ca/Tu human platelet alloantigen system. Blood 1993 (in press).

133. Kelton JG, Smith JW, Horsewood P, et al. Gov a/b alloantigen system on human platelets. Blood 1990;75:2172-6.

134. Ikeda H, Mitani T, Ohnuma M, et al. A new platelet-specific antigen, Nak^a, involved in the refractoriness of HLA-matched platelet transfusion. Vox Sang 1989;57:213-7.

135. Tomiyama Y, Take H, Ikeda H, et al. Identification of the platelet-specific alloantigen Nak^a, on platelet membrane glycoprotein IV. Blood 1990;75:684-7.

136. Yamamoto N, Ikeda H, Tandon NN, et al. A platelet membrane glycoprotein (GP) deficiency in healthy blood donors: Nak^a minus platelets lack detectable GPIV (CD36). Blood 1990; 76:1698-703.

137. Langenscheidt F, Kiefel V, Santoso S, Mueller-Eckhardt C. Platelet transfusion refractoriness associated with two rare platelet-specific alloantibodies (anti-Bak[a] and anti-Pl[A1]) and multiple HLA antibodies. Transfusion 1988;28:597-600.

138. Pamphilon DH, Farrell DH, Donaldson C, et al. Development of lymphocytotoxic and platelet reactive antibodies: A prospective study in patients with acute leukaemia. Vox Sang 1989; 57:177-81.

139. Kickler T, Kennedy SD, Braine HG. Alloimmunization to platelet-specific antigens on glycoproteins IIb-IIIa and Ib/IX in multiply transfused thrombocytopenic patients. Transfusion 1990; 30:622-5.

140. Godeau B, Fromont P, Seror T, et al. Platelet alloimmunization after multiple transfusions: A prospective study of 50 patients. Br J Haematol 1992;81:395-400.

141. Blanchette V, Chen L, Salomon DE, et al. Alloimmunization to the Pl[A1] antigen: Results of a prospective study. Br J Haematol 1990;74:209-15.

142. Reznikoff-Etievant MF, Dangu C, Lobet R. HLA-B8 antigen and anti-Pl[A1] allo-immunization. Tissue Antigens 1981;18:66-8.

143. Muller JY, Reznikoff-Etievant MF, Patereau C, Julien F. Thrombopénies néonatales par allo-immunisation à anti-Pl[A1] et antigène HLA-DR3. C R Séances Acad Sci III 1983;286:953-6.

144. Mueller-Eckhardt C, Mueller-Eckhardt G, Willen-Ohff H, et al. Immunogenicity of and immune response to the human platelet antigen Zw[a] is strongly associated with HLA-B8 and DR3. Tissue Antigens 1985;26:71-6.

145. DeWaal LP, van Dalen CM, Engelfriet CP, von dem Borne AEGKr. Alloimmunization against the platelet-specific Zw[a] antigen, resulting neonatal alloimmune thrombocytopenia or post-transfusion purpura, is associated with the supertypic DRw52 antigen including DR3 and DRw6. Hum Immunol 1986;17:45-53.

146. Mueller-Eckhardt C, Mueller-Eckhardt G. Alloimmunization against the platelet-specific Zw[a] antigen associated with HLA-DRw52 and/or DRw6? Human Immunol 1987;18:181-2.

147. Hurley CK, Gregersen PK, Gorski J, et al. The DR3(w18), DQw4 haplotype differs from DR3(w17), DQw2 haplotypes at multiple class II loci. Hum Immunol 1989;25:37-49.

148. Gorski J, Irle C, Mickelson EM, et al. Correlation of structure with T cell responses in the three members of the HLA-DRw52 allelic series. J Exp Med 1989;170:1027-32.

149. Valentin N, Vergracht A, Bignon JD, et al. HLA-DRw52a is involved in alloimmunization against Pl-A1 antigen. Hum Immunol 1990;27:73-9.

150. Decary F, L'Abbe D, Tremblay L, Chartrand P. The immune response to the HPA-1A antigen: Association with HLA-DRw52a. Transfus Med 1991;1:55-62.

151. L'Abbe D, Tremblay L, Filion M, et al. Alloimmunization to platelet antigen HPA-1A (Pl^{A1}) is strongly associated with both HLA-DRb3*0101 and HLA-DQb1*0201. Hum Immunol 1992;34: 107-14.

152. Yassai M, McFarland JG, Newton-Nash D, et al. T-cell receptor and alloimmune thrombocytopenias: A model for autoimmune diseases? Ann Intern Med 1992;143:365-70.

153. Mueller-Eckhardt C, Kiefel V, Kroll H, Mueller-Eckhardt G. HLA-DRw6, a new immune response marker for immunization against the platelet alloantigen Br^a. Vox Sang 1989;57:90-1.

154. Kuijpers RWAM, von dem Borne AEGKr, Kiefel V, et al. Leucine 33/proline 33 substitution and human platelet glycoprotein IIIa determines HLA-DRw52a (Dw24) association of the immune response against the HPA-1A (Zw^a/ Pl^{A1}) and HPA-1B (Zw^b/Pl^{A2}). Hum Immunol 1992;34:253-6.

In: Nance ST, ed.
Alloimmunity: 1993 and Beyond
Bethesda, MD: American Association of Blood Banks, 1993

5

New and Evolving Techniques for Antibody and Antigen Identification

Marilyn J. Telen, MD

S INCE DISCOVERY OF THE ABO blood groups by Landsteiner in 1900,[1] efforts to identify blood group antigens and the antibodies directed against such antibodies have become increasingly complex endeavors. Hundreds of blood group antigens have been defined by human antisera,[2] and most of them have been shown to be capable of becoming significant barriers to blood transfusion. Detection of blood group antisera and phenotyping of red cells now require significant expenditures of both reagents and technical effort.

Understanding of the biochemistry and genetics of blood group antigens has come slowly. However, we are now approaching a point in time where the biochemical and genetic bases of many major blood groups are understood.[3] We are waiting expectantly for these advances in basic science to bear fruit and improve the tools we use to deal with the day-to-day problems of transfusion—how can we more easily and more accurately identify antibody specificities, and how can we more easily and accurately identify the antigens expressed on an individual's cells?

Antigens as Epitopes

Biochemistry of Blood Group Antigens

Since the first agglutination testing was performed, a number of different methods for the detection of antigen-antibody binding have

Marilyn J. Telen, MD, Associate Professor of Medicine, Division of Hematology/Oncology, and Associate Medical Director, Transfusion Service, Duke University Medical Center, Durham, North Carolina
[This work was supported in part by grants HL 33572 and HL 44042 from the National Institutes of Health, National Heart, Lung and Blood Institute. Dr. Telen is the recipient of Research Career Development Award HL 02233 (NIH/NHLBI).]

been devised. These include radioimmunoassays[4,5] immunofluorescence assays,[6] enzyme-linked immunoassays,[7-9] as well as novel and automated methods for the detection of agglutination.[10] Several solid-phase techniques have also been developed.[11] However, the first step in devising truly new methods for antigen and antibody identification has, of necessity, been the biochemical characterization of the molecules that bear particular antigens or groups of antigens. In the case of carbohydrate antigens, such as A, B, H, Le^a, Le^b and P, the oligosaccharide structures with antigenic activity were defined relatively early, while the glycosyl-transferase proteins involved in their synthesis were characterized somewhat later. An ever-growing number of protein-dependent red blood cell group antigens have also now been localized to specific cell surface molecules (Table 5-1). However, while some of these proteins are well characterized and their functions are understood, others are known only by their molecular weights. In only a few instances do we understand the structure of the epitope involved in the expression of a particular antigen and the polymorphisms of that epitope that produce antithetical antigens.

Genetics of Blood Group Antigen Polymorphisms

Research is now extending our understanding of the biochemistry of blood group antigens to knowledge of the molecular genetic basis of antigens and their polymorphisms.[3] However, although an increasing number of cDNAs encoding blood-group-antigen-bearing molecules have been cloned, work on understanding the basis of polymorphisms has only just begun. Nevertheless, the usefulness of this knowledge has already made itself known in a wide variety of clinically important situations.

The antigens for which at least some molecular genetic information is known are listed in Table 5-2. In the case of the carbohydrate antigens, the cDNAs for several transferases have been cloned, and the differences between some transferases encoded by allelic genes have been defined. For the protein-borne antigens, a number of cDNAs encoding the proteins bearing various blood groups have been cloned, while the molecular basis of antigenic polymorphisms has been defined for only a very few blood groups.

Genetically Engineered Blood Group Antigen Expression

The ability to isolate a cDNA encoding a blood-group-antigen-bearing protein has been the first key step to envisioning a new era in antigen and antibody identification. Once a cDNA has been isolated, a number of events can take place. First, analysis of the cDNA may shed light on

Table 5-1. Biochemically Characterized Protein Blood Group Antigens

Blood Group	Protein Characteristic	Function or Significance
Rh	30-32 kD integral membrane protein	Unknown
LW	37-47 kD glycoprotein	Unknown
Duffy	35-43 kD glycoprotein	Unknown; deficiency associated with resistance to some malarial parasites
Kell	93 kD glycoprotein	Structurally part of zinc-binding metallo-proteinase family
Kx	32 kD	Unknown
Kidd	50 kD	Possibly urea transporter
MN	43 kD* integral membrane protein	Glycophorin A
'N'Ss	25 kD* integral membrane protein	Glycophorin B
Lutheran	78, 85 kD	Unknown
Xg^a	22-29 kD	Unknown
Diego	95-105 kD	Band 3 (anion transporter)
Cartwright	160 kD homodimer	Acetylcholinesterase
Scianna	60 kD	Unknown
Dombrock	47-58 kD	Unknown
In	80 kD integral membrane protein	CD44 adhesion protein
Gerbich	39 kD*	Glycophorins C and D
Gregory-Holley	47-58 kD	Possibly same as Dombrock
Cromer	70 kD phosphatidyl-inositol (PI) linked glycoprotein	Decay accelerating factor (CD55)
Ok^a	46-58 kD	Unknown
Chido/Rodgers	200 kD glycoprotein	Complement component 4 (C4)
Knops/McCoy	Variable (170-220 kD)	Complement receptor type 1 (CR1)
JMH	76 kD PI-linked glycoprotein	Unknown

*Glycophorins migrate anomalously in sodium dodecyl sulfate polyacrylamide gel electrophoresis.

Table 5-2. Blood Group Antigens for Which Molecular Genetic Information Is Known

Blood Group	cDNA Cloned	Basis of Polymorphism(s) Known
H	Yes	No
ABO	Yes	Yes
Rh	Yes	Yes
Le	Yes	No
Kell	Yes	No
MN	Yes	Yes
Ss	Yes	Yes
Diego	Yes	No
Cartwright	Yes	Yes
In	Yes	Yes
Gerbich	Yes	Yes
Cromer	Yes	Yes (some)
Chido/Rodgers	Yes	Yes (mostly)
Knops/McCoy	Yes	No

the structural orientation and function of the molecule. For example, analysis of the cDNA for the Kell protein placed it within a family of neutral zinc-binding endoproteinases that includes the CALLA antigen associated with childhood lymphoblastic leukemia.[12] In addition, hydropathy analysis enables us to predict with accuracy the orientation of a protein in the membrane—how many transmembrane segments it has, and what portions of the protein are exposed on the cell surface.[13] Then, comparison of cDNAs from individuals with different phenotypes can lead us to identification of the genetic basis of polymorphic antigens. Often, polymerase chain reaction (PCR) amplification of cDNA can accomplish such analyses in a relatively short amount of time. Identification of such genetic variation then opens up the possibility of phenotyping by genotyping—that is, determining the phenotype by analysis of the genetic sequences, either directly or indirectly, using restriction fragment length polymorphisms (RFLPs). Finally, current technology allows the creation of a DNA construct that will permit insertion and expression of the cDNA in a chosen target cell.[14] This process—called transfection—promotes the entry of foreign DNA into a eukaryotic cell and stable incorporation of the DNA into the host genome; such a transfected cell can then be grown in selection media containing a factor to which only the successfully transfected cells are resistant by virtue of a second gene, also carried by the vector. Expression of a human antigen by nonhuman cells can thus be achieved.

The advantages of using transfected cells in such a system are readily apparent when one considers the situations in which one often finds antibodies to high-incidence antigens: The blood bank has detected an antibody that makes the potential blood recipient's serum reactive with all cells in a large reagent panel. The patient may or may not have other previously identified alloantibodies to complicate the picture. Thus, the technologist is wondering: Does the fact that all cells are reactive mean that there are multiple antibodies, or is it one antibody that is against a high-incidence antigen? To answer that question, the technologist has several choices. He or she may try to determine something about the nature of the target antibody by using enzyme-treated cells. If that fails to indicate the presence of multiple antibodies whose antigens have varying enzyme sensitivity or to narrow down the list of possible antigen targets due to the sensitivity pattern, the technologist must face a two-fold chore. If available, phenotypically rare red cells must be obtained from the freezer for testing with the patient's serum. If the patient has more than one alloantibody, these cells must fail to express those antigens already identified as antibody targets. In addition, the technologist may need rare sera from the freezer to do an extensive phenotype of the patient's cells. This process will be further complicated if the patient has been transfused and no pretransfusion cells are available for testing.

Now think how simple things would be if the technologist could obtain from the freezer or refrigerator a selection of cells, each one of which expressed only one common blood group antigen. How could this be done? In theory, quite simply! First, a nonhuman cell line bearing no human blood groups could be selected, grown in quantity and prepared for transfection. Separate aliquots could then be transfected with specific cDNA-containing vectors, each expressing a single blood group antigen molecule. These aliquots can then be grown and expanded into immortal cell lines, each expressing only one blood group antigen. So, when the technologist is faced with an antibody either to a high-incidence antigen or in the setting of multiple antibodies, the puzzle could be quickly solved using easily available and replaceable cells, each bearing only one blood group antigen.

At least one problem remains, however: What method would we want to use to test for reactivity with nucleated, and possibly adherent, transfected cells? Clearly, we would want a method that required minimal expensive equipment and that was reliable, reproducible and readily learned. Thus far, a number of methods have been used. These include agglutination inhibition by adsorption of antibody onto transfected cells, immunofluorescent flow cytometric assay, Western blot, dot blot and agglutination inhibition using specially prepared extracts of transfected cells. The following discussion illustrates how some methods of analyzing DNA or recombinant antigens have been used in both clinical and research situations.

Making Sense of ABO

The recent progress in the ABO system illustrates how some of these new techniques can help in the identification and understanding of phenotypes within a blood group system. After cloning the cDNA for the blood group A N-acetylgalactosaminyl transferase,[15] Yamamoto, Hakomori and their colleagues set about to determine the molecular basis of the other ABO phenotypes. Analysis of cDNA from group O individuals all showed a simple single base pair deletion (nucleotide 258, when position 1 is the beginning of the initiation codon) that caused a shift in the reading frame and, shortly thereafter, a premature stop codon.[16] Thus, the O gene was similar to the A gene except for a single mutation that led to the inability to express a complete transferase molecule. The gene from group B individuals, however, showed more complex differences. Instead of a single change, B genes from several individuals differed from their A counterparts at four bases distributed over a coding region of 1065 base pairs.[16] These nucleotide polymorphisms lead to amino acid substitutions at positions 176, 235, 266 and 268. How many of these were involved in the change of substrate specificity from N-acetyl galactosamine to galactose? To answer this question, these researchers went through the laborious process of making DNA constructs representing all possible combinations containing the bases present in the A and B genes.[17] Each construct was then transfected into and expressed by HeLa cells in culture, so that these cells could be tested for transferase activity and for transferase substrate specificity. The results, shown in Table 5-3, demonstrate that it is possible to produce transferases with a variety of specificities. Some could form A or B structures with equal ease (AB transferases), while others formed predominantly or only one or the other blood group antigen. Thus, a single series of well-thought-out experiments showed that at least three of the four base pair changes contribute to transferase substrate specificity and, in addition, demonstrated possible causes of several unusual phenotypes, including cis AB, B(A) and A(B). Indeed, more recently, a cis AB phenotype has been proven to be the result of two mutations of the A_1 gene[18]: the first is a single base pair mutation associated with the A_2 phenotype,[19] while the second is a base pair substitution that matches one of the four associated with the B phenotype. Thus, this single variant gene produces an AB phenotype with A_2-like A expression and B_3-like B antigen expression.

This study of ABO genes brings us to the realization that we can now apply new techniques to ABO typing. First, we can use RFLP analysis to identify nucleotide substitutions associated with various ABO phenotypes.[16,20] Although from a practical standpoint it is most often easier to type cells serologically, we can imagine instances in which serologic results are confusing or unavailable. After massive transfusion, there may no longer be any patient's red cells to type if a

Table 5-3. A-B Transferase Activity Is Dependent on the Amino Acids Present at Various Positions in the Recombinant Transferase Protein

Amino Acids Present (position #)				Transferase Activity
#176	#235	#266	#268	
A	A	A	A	A
A	A	A	B	A
A	A	B	A	AB
A	A	B	B	B
A	B	A	A	A
A	B	A	B	A(B)
A	B	B	A	AB
A	B	B	B	B
B	A	A	A	A
B	A	A	B	A
B	A	B	A	AB
B	A	B	B	B
B	B	A	A	A
B	B	A	B	A(B)
B	B	B	A	AB
B	B	B	B	B

(Adapted from Yamamoto and Hakomori.[17])

question arises. After bone marrow transplant, circulating blood cells may be of donor origin; in that case, other cellular material can be used as a source of DNA. And, in the case of unusual inheritance patterns, such as cis AB, genetic evidence may explain unusual serologic findings. In all these instances, the patient's true antigenic phenotype may be more clearly understood by investigation of the genotype.

RFLP Analysis of PCR Products

Use of PCR in RFLP analysis can potentially be applied to many areas, including phenotyping of platelets. Rather than digest total genomic DNA, a process that produces a smear of variably sized DNA fragments, PCR amplification produces a single amplification product, usually of constant size, irrespective of the polymorphism present, such as ABO. These amplification products can then be subjected to restriction enzyme digestion and analysis by gel electrophoresis. Products of digestion can then be stained in the gel with ethidium bromide and visualized directly under UV light. Photographic records can be easily made for documentation and review of data. This process is faster than standard RFLP analysis by Southern blotting and does not require tedious labeling of gene-specific probes, transfer of DNA fragments to nitrocellulose or nylon membranes, nucleic acid hybridization of probes, washing and either exposure to film or development of a colored substrate in enzyme-linked methods of detection. Instead, DNA is prepared and amplified by PCR. The product is digested in a few hours, and within a few more hours at most, the results are apparent.

ABO Genotyping by Allele-Specific RFLP Analysis

The human *O* transferase gene differs from the *A* gene by a single nucleotide deletion, loss of the G at nucleotide position 258 (with nucleotide position 1 being the beginning of the initiation codon).[16] This change destroys a BstEII site and, at the same time, creates a new KpnI site (Fig 5-1). When the KpnI site is present in the *O* gene, a fragment smaller than that found in *A* and *B* genes can be identified by Southern blotting using a probe including a large nonpolymorphic stretch of DNA. Likewise, in an *A* or *B* gene, the presence of the BstEII site produces a restriction fragment 3 kb smaller than that found in the PCR product from *O* genes.

The B transferase differs from its A counterpart at four positions, amino acids 176, 235, 266 and 268.[16] The first three of these substitutions result from nucleotide changes that also cause alteration in restriction enzyme recognition sites, in each instance destroying a restriction site normally present in the *A* and *O* genes as well as creating a new restriction site typical of the *B* gene. These can easily be seen after restriction enzyme digestion of PCR products, without DNA hybridization. Thus, PCR products from *A* and *O* genes will give rise to a 262 base pair NarI fragment, while similar products from *B* genes will give rise to a 205 bp NarI fragment (Fig 5-1). Differences can also be detected using BssHII, which detects a recognition site in *A* and *O* genes that overlaps with the NarI site detected in *B* genes, as well as HpaII and AluI, which identify overlapping sites present or absent, respectively, in *A* and *O* vs *B* genes. Using this type of analysis, Lee and Chang have successfully ABO-grouped numerous types of samples, including peripheral blood samples as well as forensic samples of saliva stains, semen stains, hair and bone tissue.[20] Other investigators have used these techniques to resolve the question of whether the patient was of the genetic or acquired B phenotype. Again, RFLP analysis of PCR products allowed determination that no *B* gene was present, thus proving the blood group genotype independently of the expression of blood group antigen molecules.[21]

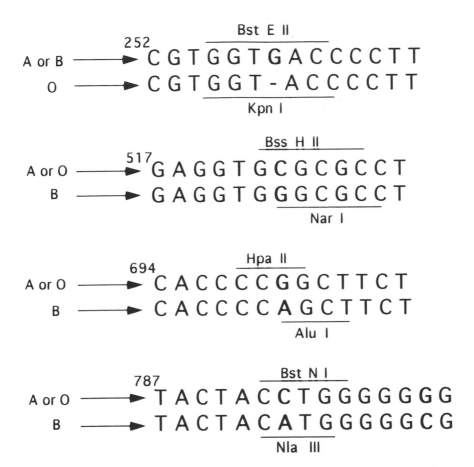

Figure 5-1. ABO genotyping by allele-specific RFLP analysis. Both the single nucleotide deletion found in the *O* gene and three of the four nucleotide substitutions that differentiate *A* from *B* genes can be identified via RFLP analysis. The variation in BstEII and KpnI digestion products can be seen by standard Southern blotting; with both these enzymes, the *O* gene pattern differs from that shared by *A* and *B* genes. RFLP analysis to differentiate *A* from *B* genes is most easily done by digestion of PCR products. (Adapted from Yamamoto et al.[16])

Use of Transfectants in Identifying Rare Blood Group Antibodies

When a patient needing a transfusion has made an antibody to a high-incidence antigen, identification of the antibody specificity and subsequent localization of antigen-negative blood may consume an inordinate amount of technologist time and rare reagents, and may also delay transfusion to the point of threatening the well-being of the patient. In 1988, the Cromer blood group antigens were shown to reside on a membrane protein called decay accelerating factor, or DAF.[22] Soon thereafter, the Cromer null—or Inab—phenotype was found to result from the lack of expression of DAF.[23] Since the DAF cDNA and gene structure were known a short time later,[24] this system became an early model for investigating how biochemical and molecular techniques might be applied to the identification of antigens and antibodies.

Allele-Specific Transfectants

The first polymorphism within the Cromer blood group to be investigated at the molecular level was Dr(a–).[25] Analysis of genomic sequences showed a single base pair mutation in the exon encoding the latter half of the third so-called short consensus repeat of DAF. This mutation caused a single amino acid substitution, serine to leucine at amino acid 165. That this mutation was responsible for the antigenic phenotype—Dr(a-)—was shown by using allele-specific transfectants.[25] Cell lines expressing either normal cDNA or a DNA sequence mutated to contain the Dr(a–)-type mutation were tested by a variety of methods for Dr^a antigen expression. One method, familiar to serologists, is that of adsorption. Three types of cells were used: cells carrying vector DNA without the DAF sequence, cells carrying the vector with the DAF sequence and cells carrying the vector with the mutated DAF sequence. When these three types of cells were used to adsorb anti-Dr^a, only one cell line was active—the cells expressing the normal DAF cDNA sequence. When anti-DAF murine monoclonal and rabbit polyclonal antibodies were tested by immunofluorescence, however, two cell lines reacted: the cells expressing the normal DAF sequence and the cells expressing the mutated DAF sequence (Fig 5-2). The cells carrying only vector DAF did not react with anti-DAF. Thus, parallel results were obtained using flow cytometry and adsorption/inhibition. The single base pair change did not impair expression of other DAF epitopes but did prevent reactivity with anti-Dr^a.

Since those studies, additional methods of using transfectants have been explored. One of the more common Cromer antibodies is against the Cr^a antigen. The molecular basis of that epitope has also been worked out and shown to be a G to C substitution in the fourth consensus repeat, leading to a proline-to-alanine substitution in that area (Telen MJ et al, unpublished observations). Again, an allele-specific transfectant was made containing that single mutation. As expected, multiple antisera against Cr^a failed to react with the transfectant cells carrying this point mutation.

Next, attempts were made to establish an easy, solid-phase technology that could utilize this ability to make allele-specific transfectants. Nondenaturing detergent lysates were made from the transfectant cells expressing normal DAF, Dr(a–) DAF and Cr(a–) DAF. Similar

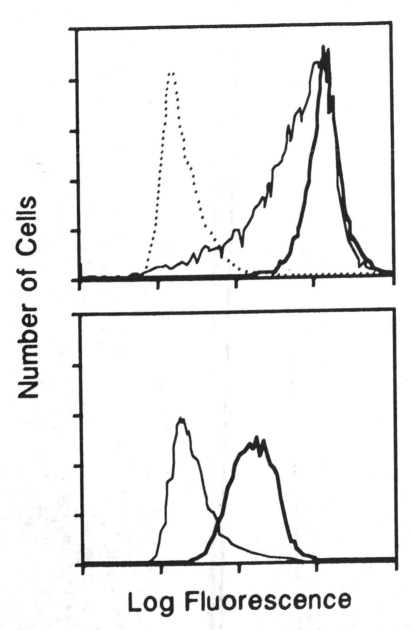

Figure 5-2. Immunofluorescence flow cytometric analysis of allele-specific transfectants bearing Cromer blood group antigens. CHO cells transfected with vector only (dotted line), wild-type Dr(a+) DAF cDNA (thick line) or variant cDNA containing the point mutation found in Dr(a−) individuals (thin line) reacted with rabbit anti-DAF (upper panel) or human anti-Dr[a] (lower panel). Transfection with both the wild-type and variant DAF cDNAs resulted in high DAF expression; however, only cells containing the wild-type DAF cDNA reacted with anti-Dr[a]. (Reprinted with permission from Lublin et al.[25])

lysates were also made from red cell membrane preparations. Small aliquots of these lysates—only 5-10 µL—were then pipetted onto nitrocellulose strips. These strips were then incubated first in human sera with or without Cromer blood group specificities. After washing, reactivity was visualized using an alkaline phosphatase-linked anti-human globulin reagent. Results showed unequivocal concordance with routine serology. As shown in Fig 5-3, anti-Cr^a reacted with the normal DAF and with the Dr(a−) DAF but not with the Cr(a−) DAF expressed by the transfected cells. Likewise, anti-Dr^a reacted with all but the Dr(a−) transfectants.

For this antigenic system, the dot blot method is easily accomplished. Nitrocellulose sheets to which membrane proteins have been attached can potentially be stored for long periods without appreciable loss of antigenicity. Or, frozen cell lysates can be stored for months to years and then thawed and applied to nitrocellulose without any

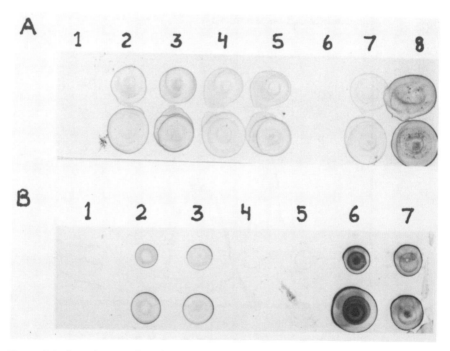

Figure 5-3. Assaying transfected cells with human alloantibody using dot blot. In Panel A, anti-Cr^a was reacted with nitrocellulose containing extracts of CHO cells expressing various DNA constructs: 1) vector only, 2) normal DAF cDNA, 3) DAF with SCR1 (short consensus repeat 1) deleted, 4) DAF with SCR2 deleted, 5) DAF with SCR3 deleted, 6) DAF with SCR4 deleted, 7) DAF with the Ser/Thr-rich segment deleted and 8) Cr(a+) red cells. In Panel B, anti-Cr^a was reacted with extracts of CHO cells expressing 1) vector only, 2) normal DAF cDNA, 3) DAF with SCR3 deleted, 4) DAF with SCR4 deleted, 5) DAF with the Cr(a−) type of change in SCR4, 6) DAF with the Dr(a−) type of change in SCR3 and 7) Cr(a+) Dr(a+) red cells.

high-technology equipment. Analogous methods are also probably practicable using enzyme-linked immunosorbent assay (ELISA) technology, in which the cell lysate is attached to the bottom of plastic wells, and color change of the indicator enzyme-linked antiglobulin reagent is measured by an ELISA reader.

Usefulness of Deletion Transfectants

Note also that one does not need to have identified the biochemical and genetic basis for a polymorphism to identify an antibody by this technique. For example, Lublin and colleagues have created a series of deletion mutations in DAF cDNA, each of which is missing one of the five protein domains.[26] Each mutant DAF cDNA was inserted via an appropriate vector into host cells and expressed by a transfected cell line. When these cell lines were tested with anti-Dr^a and anti-Cr^a, the DAF mutant cell lines reacted with the antibodies except when the specific epitope was disturbed by the mutation (Fig 5-3). Thus, anti-Cr^a reacted with all lines but the one missing the fourth consensus repeat. Anti-Dr^a reacted with all lines except those missing the third or fourth consensus repeats. This result indicates that, although the mutation creating the Dr(a–) phenotype occurs in the third consensus repeat, the fourth repeat is also necessary for expression of the Dr^a epitope. Such a system of deletion mutants could potentially be used to screen antibodies to high-incidence antigens within the Cromer blood group. Cromer specificity would be confirmed by reactivity with cells carrying transfected DAF cDNA but not with cells carrying vector only. Use of deletion mutants could then determine epitope location. Once all the known Cromer antigens are mapped, the pattern of reactivity with such mutants would also indicate which Cromer antigen was likely to be the antibody target. Confirmation could then be accomplished using an allele-specific transfectant.

The MN System: Sorting Out the Antigens and Antibodies

Work in the 1970's led to the identification of glycophorin A as the protein bearing the M and N antigens[27,28] and a paired amino acid substitution at positions 1 and 5 of glycophorin A as the basis for the MN polymorphism.[29-31] Since that time, much genetic information has been obtained concerning the glycophorin A gene, the highly related glycophorin B gene and a third gene—thus far unassociated with blood group antigen activity—glycophorin E.[32] In addition, we now know the gene structure of many glycophorin variants,[33-35] termed

Miltenberger types, and this has led to an understanding of the antigens expressed by these cells.

What Do Anti-M and Anti-N Recognize?

Once the structures of the M and N determinants were identified and cDNAs encoding these glycophorin A isoforms were cloned, we first became truly able to decipher the real specificities of M and N antibodies. In a simple but elegant study, both murine monoclonal antibodies as well as human anti-M were assayed for their specificities.[36] The researchers used the technique of making transfectant cell lines that expressed glycophorin cDNAs. By the technique of site-directed mutagenesis, four DNA sequences were created (Fig 5-4).[36] The first two had the sequences characteristic of the M or N variant of glycophorin A, encoding either serine and glycine or leucine and glutamine in amino acid positions 1 and 5. The third encoded serine at the first amino acid position, like M, but glutamine at the fifth position, like N. This variant corresponds to the M^c phenotype. The fourth sequence represented the opposite type of construct, with leucine at the first position, like N, but glycine at the fifth position, like M. This variant has not been described. When a murine monoclonal anti-M antibody was tested with these various constructs, it required presence of the glycine at position 5, but not the serine at position 1, and thus reacted with the normal M-type glycophorin as well as the leucine/glycine combination thus far not known to occur naturally; it also required presence of the normal sialic residues at the N-terminus. However, three examples of human anti-M required the serine at

	Genetically engineered MN variant	Murine anti-M	Human anti-M	Vicea graminea	Murine anti-N
M:	NH$_2$-Ser-Ser-Thr-Thr-Gly-R	+	+	—	—
M^c:	NH$_2$-Ser-Ser-Thr-Thr-Glu-R	—	+	—	—
N:	NH$_2$-Leu-Ser-Thr-Thr-Glu-R	—	—	+	+
	NH$_2$-Leu-Ser-Thr-Thr-Gly-R	+	—	+	+

Figure 5-4. Site-directed mutation analysis of M and N specificity. CHO cells were used to express the four possible combinations of ser/leu and gly/glu substitutions at amino acid positions 1 and 5, respectively. Extracts of these cells were then tested for M and N antigenic activity, using a variety of reagents. No reagent tested required both amino acid substitutions for recognition of the M or N antigens. (Adapted from Blackall et al.[36])

position 1, while the glycine at position 5 was not essential. Thus, although equivalent in most practical situations, the murine and human antibodies did not recognize the same epitopes and could provide misleading or contradictory results in special circumstances.

Investigation of the specificity of anti-N antibodies was more difficult. The N-lectin *Vicea graminea* was shown to require the leucine at position 1 but not the glutamine at position 5.[36] However, multiple samples of human anti-N failed to react with the appropriate transfected cells, demonstrating that—despite the correct amino acid sequence—other factors, such as glycosylation, were able to interfere with the expression of the N epitope.[37]

Allele-Specific Oligonucleotide Primers

Because the MN-glycophorin A system is among the best understood, it has been the target of attempts to apply other DNA-based technologies as well. Recently, a group of investigators has shown that a rapid PCR method can be used to MN phenotype individuals accurately and with minimal samples.[38] Using this technique, workers targeted the polymorphic N-terminal region of glycophorin A for amplification. By running two reactions for each sample, with each reaction using a primer containing the M- or N-type sequence at one end and a common primer at the other, they were able to show that detectable amplification would occur only when the primer sequence matched the sequence of the target DNA. Thus, in heterozygotes, both reactions would produce amplified DNA, while in homozygotes, only the reaction with the appropriate primer would be productive. Analysis could be accomplished quickly by agar gel electrophoresis. Moreover, as little as 0.5-1.0 µg whole blood was required for each reaction, and the technique is easy to apply to large numbers of samples when necessary, as perhaps in forensic analysis or population or linkage studies. A somewhat similar allele-specific PCR technique has also been used for typing in the ABO system.[39] In that system, a single reaction for each sample contains four primer sets. The size of the products depends on which primers are active, according to genotype.

Allele-specific PCR can be more useful than RFLP analysis with or without PCR for several reasons. First, analysis of genomic DNA without PCR necessitates knowledge of RFLP variants that occur independently of blood group polymorphisms. When a particular enzyme is associated with RFLP variants that depend on noncoding region polymorphisms, for example, family studies may be required to sort out which bands are the result of polymorphisms in introns and which are the result of the exonic polymorphisms that determine blood group-related genotype. Second, allele-specific PCR has an advantage over RFLP analysis of PCR products because no second step is required. The PCR products can be definitively analyzed by gel electrophoresis without first accomplishing restriction enzyme digestion.

The Miltenberger Phenotypes: Usefulness of Synthetic Peptides

Perhaps the greatest contribution of this new technology has been the attainment of an accurate understanding of the Miltenberger phenotypes. Analysis of the genes responsible for these phenotypes has finally explained how many of these genes arise as well as what the antibodies directed toward them react with. In the last few years, many of the Miltenberger glycophorin variants have undergone extensive biochemical and genetic examination. Out of this work has come important insights into the serology of the Miltenberger antigens and antibodies.

The amino acid sequences that form the basis of the Mur, Hil and Hop specificities have been determined by analysis of the genes encoding MiIII, MiV, MiJ.L., MiVI and MiVIII glycophorin variants.[34] Although Mur and Hil occur together on MiIII and MiVI red cells, this work has shown that they recognize different peptides. The Hil peptide sequence occurs in MiV cells, in which a glycophorin A/B hybrid is expressed; in these cells, the peptide surrounding the A/B junction expresses the Hil epitope. In MiIII cells, however, a glycophorin B/A/B hybrid is expressed. The Hil antigen again occurs at the A/B junction. However, the Mur antigen occurs within a peptide closer to the N-terminal, encoded by the glycophorin B pseudoexon that is expressed in the rearranged MiIII gene. A similar peptide sequence is expressed by the MiVI gene, which also encodes a glycophorin B/A/B hybrid with a different B/A junction.

Knowledge of the sequence of these variant glycophorins has been used to design epitope-specific peptides expressing the Hil, Hop and Mur antigens (Fig 5-5).[34] In each case, one or more antisera could be shown to be inhibited from agglutinating antigen-positive cells by the specific peptide. Thus, if it turns out to be the case that most antibodies with these specificities are relatively independent of the secondary structure that might only exist within the intact glycophorin molecule, we can reasonably plan to equip at least our reference laboratories with the peptides that can help us identify antibodies to these unusual antigens. These peptides might be useful as inhibitors of agglutination, and thus serve to identify antibody specificity, or they might be supplied immobilized on a solid matrix, for measurement of reactivity via enzyme-linked antibody binding.

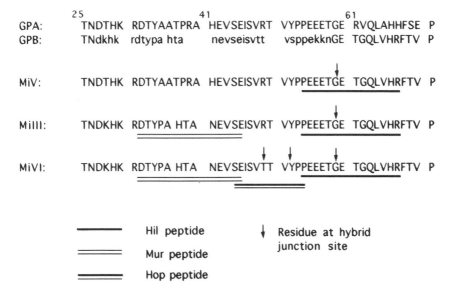

Figure 5-5. Peptide sequences that carry the rare blood group antigens Hil, Mur and Hop. The normal and variant amino acid sequences of normal glycophorin A (GPA), glycophorin B (GPB) and the Miltenberger variants MiV, MiIII and MiVI have been deduced from cDNA sequences and are expressed in standard one-letter code. (Upper case indicates expressed codons, while lower case indicates normally unexpressed codons that are part of the GPB pseudoexon.) The underlined peptides have inhibitory activity for antibodies directed to the antigens indicated. Arrows indicate putative junctions of the rearranged GPA and GPB genes. (Adapted from Johe et al.[34])

Diagnosis of Clinically Important Null Phenotypes by Biochemical and DNA Technologies

Several null blood group phenotypes are of clinical significance. For example, the Rh_{null} phenotype is associated with chronic low-grade hemolytic anemia.[40] Diagnosis of this phenotype is relatively easy, however, because antisera to the five major Rh antigens are commonly available and quite reliable. However, mild chronic hemolytic anemia can also be associated with the Leach phenotype, a cause—albeit unusual—of hereditary elliptocytosis.[41] The Leach phenotype is the null phenotype in the Gerbich blood group system,[42] and the Gerbich antigens are carried by glycophorin C.[43] However, not all cells that are Ge-negative have the Leach phenotype. Most Ge:–2,–3 cells express a variant glycophorin C molecule that fails to express Gerbich antigens but nevertheless functions well in its role as an attachment site for cytoskeletal protein.[44] Thus, distinguishing between the Ge: –2,–3 and Leach phenotypes is difficult. Initial discrimination was accomplished by protein gel electrophoresis, as well as by patterns of reactivity with

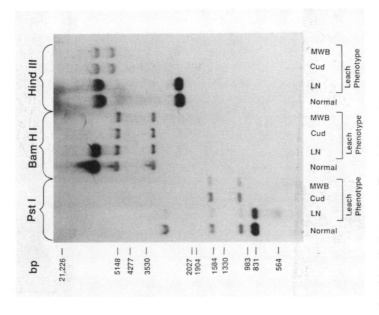

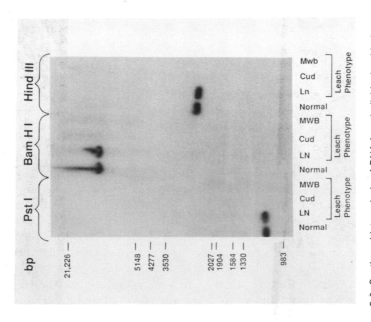

Figure 5-6. Southern blot analysis of DNA from individuals with the normal (Ge+) and Leach phenotypes. Two of three individuals who failed to express Gerbich antigens and glycophorin C (GPC) on their red cells (Leach phenotype) lack genomic DNA corresponding to exons 3 and 4 of the GPC gene. In Panel A, genomic DNA digested with the indicated enzymes was hybridized with a complete cDNA probe; in Panel B, a probe specific for exon 4 was used. (Reprinted with permission from Telen et al.[47])

monoclonal antibodies that react with both the normal and variant forms of glycophorin C.[45] Investigation of the molecular basis of the Leach phenotype has revealed that most cases are due to deletion of the genetic material comprising two exons of the glycophorin C gene (Fig 5-6).[46,47] This then opens the way for rapid diagnosis of this phenotype by PCR or dot blot techniques, using probes or primers specific for the genetic material deleted in the Leach phenotype.

Where Do We Go From Here?

Since the early descriptions of the technique for producing hybridomas, we have moved relatively quickly into the clinical use of numerous monoclonal antibody reagents. These reagents are essentially endlessly reproducible and, theoretically at least, should maintain constant characteristics indefinitely. Along the way, however, we have learned that they do not always act like our old reagents. So we have discovered that some B cells will phenotype as AB with certain monoclonal reagents. And some monoclonal antiglobulin reagents have narrower reactivity than did the polyclonal reagents we used to use. But we have adapted and learned. In recompense, these reagents are no longer of human origin and, presumably, have less propensity to be infectious for the technologists working with them. Their characteristics should prove more constant and reliable in the long run. In the case of antiglobulin reagents, we can know definitively what specificities the antibodies have, such as what complement components or breakdown products will be reactive.

We are now at the beginning of the road leading to technical advances based not on monoclonal antibody technology, but on molecular genetics. In the HLA field, new serologic specificities will now be required to correlate with a specific allelic DNA sequence.[48] In other words, serologic reactivity will no longer be considered enough to define an allele or an antigen. In that sense, we may have more work to do, not less. Ultimately, however, these advances in the genetics of antigens should make our lives as blood bankers easier. If an antibody arises in a heavily transfused patient, we will no longer need to painstakingly isolate reticulocytes for phenotyping; instead, a few drops of peripheral blood containing leukocytes will provide the DNA necessary for genotyping in the blood group system of interest. Then, to resolve which antibodies we are detecting, we will be able to obtain from the refrigerator the genetically engineered reagents—cells or extracts immobilized on a solid-phase matrix—needed to identify the specificities of the antibodies detected. The technologist will be able to select these reagents on the basis of the single expressed blood group antigen and not have to worry about what antigens of other blood group systems are also expressed. And, when high-incidence antigens appear to be the problem, the technologist will not have to search for the rare cells in the laboratory freezer and be concerned about using the last of them. Recombinant reagents will be endlessly available because they will be derived from immortal cell lines. Also, the issue of whether such reagents carry infectious diseases will no longer be important. So far, these methodologies are still in the research and development phase. However, there is little doubt that during the next decade they will gradually replace at least some of the techniques we are using now.

Acknowledgments

The author thanks Dr. Douglas Lublin for his collaboration in and contributions to joint work on the Cromer blood group system and Drs. Jean-Pierre Cartron, Yves Colin and Caroline Le Van Kim for providing a first practical introduction to molecular genetics.

References

1. Landsteiner K. Über Agglutinationserscheinungen normalen menschlichen Blutes. Wien Klin Wochenschr 1901;14:1132-4.
2. Issitt PD. Applied blood group serology. 3rd ed. Miami: Montgomery Scientific Publications, 1985.
3. Lutz P, Dzik WH. Molecular biology of red cell blood group genes. Transfusion 1992;32:467-83.
4. Chow SF, Telen MJ, Rosse WF. The acetylcholinesterase defect in paroxysmal nocturnal hemoglobinuria: Evidence that the enzyme is absent from the cell membrane. Blood 1985;66:940-5.
5. Nilsson Ekdahl K, Loof L, Nilsson UR, Nilsson B. Development of an immunoassay for the detection of minute amounts of IgG-coated erythrocytes in whole blood and its application for the assessment of Fc-mediated clearance of anti-D coated erythrocytes in vivo. Vox Sang 1989;57:188-92.
6. Nance ST. Application of flow cytometry in blood transfusion science. In: Moore SB, ed. Progress in immunohematology. Arlington, VA: American Association of Blood Banks, 1988:1-30.
7. Riley JZ, Ness PM, Taddie SJ, et al. Detection and quantitation of fetal maternal hemorrhage utilizing an enzyme-linked antiglobulin test. Transfusion 1982;22:472-4.
8. Kickler TS, Smith B, Bell W, et al. Estimation of transfused cell survival using an enzyme-linked antiglobulin test. Transfusion 1985;25:401-5.

9. Greenwalt TJ, Dumuswala UJ, Siongco A, Domino MM. An enzyme-linked antibody test to detect red cell globulins after glutaraldehyde fixation. Vox Sang 1992;63:262-7.

10. Lapierre Y, Rigal D, Adam J, et al. The gel test: A new way to detect red cell antigen-antibody reactions. Transfusion 1990;30: 109-13.

11. Sinor LT. Advances in solid phase red cell adherence methods and transfusion serology. Transfus Med Rev 1992;6:26-31.

12. Lee S, Zambas E, Marsh WL, Redman CM. Molecular cloning and primary structure of Kell blood group protein. Proc Natl Acad Sci USA 1991;88:6353-7.

13. Hartmann E, Rapoport TA, Lodish HF. Predicting the orientation of eukaryotic membrane spanning proteins. Proc Natl Acad Sci USA 1989;86:5786-90.

14. Elder JT, Spritz RA, Weissman SM. Simian virus 40 as a eukaryotic cloning vehicle. Annu Rev Genet 1981;15:295-340.

15. Yamamoto F, Marken J, Tsuji T, et al. Cloning and characterization of DNA complementary to human UDP-GalNAc:Fuc 1-2Gal 1-3GalNAc transferase (histo-blood group A transferase) mRNA. J Biol Chem 1990;265:1146-51.

16. Yamamoto F, Clausen H, White T, et al. Molecular genetic basis of the histo-blood group ABO system. Nature 1990;345:229-33.

17. Yamamoto F, Hakomori S. Sugar-nucleotide donor specificity of histo-blood group A and B transferases is based on amino acid substitutions. J Biol Chem 1990;265:19257-52.

18. Yamamoto F, McNeill PD, Kominato Y, et al. Molecular genetic analysis of the ABO blood group system: (II) Cis AB alleles. Vox Sang 1993;64:120-3.

19. Yamamoto F, McNeill PD, Hakomori S. Human histo-blood group A_2 transferase coded by A_2 allele, one of the A subtypes, is characterized by a single base deletion in the coding sequence, which results in an additional domain at the carboxyl terminal. Biochem Biophys Res Commun 1992;187:366-74.

20. Lee JC, Chang JG. ABO genotyping by polymerase chain reaction. J Forensic Sci 1992;37:1269-75.

21. Fischer GF, Fae I, Dub E, Pickl WF. Analysis of the gene polymorphism of ABO blood group specific transferases helps diagnosis of acquired B status. Vox Sang 1992;62:113-6.

22. Telen MJ, Hall SE, Green AM, et al. Identification of human erythrocyte blood group antigens on decay-accelerating factor (DAF) and an erythrocyte phenotype negative for DAF. J Exp Med 1988;167:1993-8.

23. Telen MJ, Green AM. The Inab phenotype: Characterization of the membrane protein and complement regulatory defect. Blood 1989;74:437-41.

24. Post TW, Arce MA, Liszewski MK, et al. Structure of the gene for human complement protein decay accelerating factor. J Immunol 1990;144:740-4.
25. Lublin DM, Thompson EM, Green AM, et al. Dr(a–) polymorphism of decay accelerating factor. Biochemical, functional and molecular characterization and production of allele-specific transfectants. J Clin Invest 1991;87:1945-52.
26. Coyne KE, Hall SE, Thompson ES, et al. Mapping of epitopes, glycosylation sites, and complement regulatory domains in human decay accelerating factor. J Immunol 1992;149:2906-13.
27. Hamaguchi H, Cleve H. Solubilization of human erythrocyte membrane glycoproteins and separation of the MN glycoprotein from a glycoprotein with I, S, and A activity. Biochim Biophys Acta 1972;278:271-80.
28. Tomita M, Marchesi VT. Amino acid sequence and oligosaccharide attachment sites of human erythrocyte glycophorin. Proc Natl Acad Sci USA 1975;72:2964-8.
29. Dahr W, Uhlenbruck G, Janssen E, Schmalisch R. Different N-terminal amino acids in the M,N glycoprotein from MM and NN erythrocytes. Hum Genet 1977;35:335-43.
30. Wasniowska K, Drzeniek Z, Lisowska E. The amino acids of M and N blood group glycopeptides are different. Biochem Biophys Res Commun 1977;76:385-90.
31. Furthmayr H. Structural comparison of glycophorins and immunochemical analysis of genetic variants. Nature 1978;271:519-24.
32. Cartron JP, London J. The protein and gene structure of red cell glycophorins. In: Agre PC, Cartron JP, eds. Protein blood group antigens of the human red cell: Structure, function, and significance. Baltimore, MD: Johns Hopkins University Press, 1992:101-51.
33. Huang CH, Spruell P, Moulds JJ, Blumenfeld OO. Molecular basis for the human erythrocyte glycophorin specifying the Miltenberger Class I (MiI) phenotype. Blood 1992;80:257-63.
34. Johe KK, Vengelen-Tyler V, Leger R, Blumenfeld OO. Synthetic peptides homologous to human glycophorins of the Miltenberger complex of variants of MNSs blood group system specify the epitopes for Hil, SJL, Hop, and Mur antisera. Blood 1991;78:2456-61.
35. Huang CH, Blumenfeld OO. Molecular genetics of human erythrocyte MiIII and MiVI glycophorins: Use of a pseudoexon in construction of two delta-alpha-delta hybrid genes resulting in antigenic diversification. J Biol Chem 1991;266:7248-55.
36. Blackall DP, Ugorski M, Pahlsson P, Spitalnik SL. Determination of the fine specificity of antigen-antibody interactions using mutants of recombinant glycophorin A (abstract). Transfusion 1992; 32:24S.

37. Blackall DP, Ugorski M, Smith ME, et al. The binding of human alloantibodies to recombinant glycophorin A. Transfusion 1992; 32:629-32.
38. Corfield VA, Moolman JC, Martell R, Brink PA. Polymerase chain reaction-based detection of MN blood group-specific sequences in the human genome. Transfusion 1993;33:119-24.
39. Ugozzoli L, Wallace RB. Application of an allele-specific polymerase chain reaction to the direct determination of ABO blood group genotypes. Genomics 1992;12:670-4.
40. Nash R, Shojania AM. Hematological aspect of Rh deficiency syndrome: A case report and review of the literature. Am J Hematol 1987;24:267-75.
41. Anstee DJ, Parsons SF, Ridgwell K, et al. Two individuals with elliptocytic red cells lack three minor erythrocyte membrane sialoglycoproteins. Biochem J 1984;221:97-104.
42. Daniels GL, Shaw MA, Judson PA, et al. A family demonstrating inheritance of the Leach phenotype: A Gerbich-negative phenotype associated with elliptocytosis. Vox Sang 1986;50:117-21.
43. Dahr W, Kiedrowski S, Blanchard D, et al. High frequency antigens of human erythrocyte membrane sialoglycoproteins. V. Characterization of the Gerbich blood group antigens: Ge2 and Ge3. Biol Chem Hoppe Seyler 1987;368:1375-83.
44. Dahr W, Moulds J, Baumeister G, et al. Altered membrane sialoglycoproteins in human erythrocytes lacking the Gerbich blood group antigens. Biol Chem Hoppe Seyler 1985;366:201-11.
45. Dahr W, Blanchard D, Kiedrowski S, et al. High frequency antigens of human erythrocyte membrane sialoglycoproteins. VI. Monoclonal antibodies reacting with the N-terminal domain of glycophorin C. Biol Chem Hoppe Seyler 1989;370:849-54.
46. Tanner MJA, High S, Martin PG, et al. Genetic variants of human red cell membrane sialoglycoprotein beta: Study of the alterations occurring in the sialoglycoprotein beta gene. Biochem J 1988;250:407-14.
47. Telen MJ, Le Van Kim C, Ching A, et al. Molecular basis for elliptocytosis associated with glycophorin C and D deficiency in the Leach phenotype. Blood 1991;78:1603-6.
48. Bodmer JG, Marsh SGE, Albert ED, et al. Nomenclature for factors in the HLA system. Hum Immunol 1991;34:4-18.

In: Nance ST, ed.
Alloimmunity: 1993 and Beyond
Bethesda, MD: American Association of Blood Banks, 1993

6

New Insights Into the Pathophysiology and Treatment of Acute Hemolytic Transfusion Reactions

Stephen M. Capon, MD, and Dennis Goldfinger, MD

TRANSFUSIONS OF BLOOD AND blood components have increased tremendously in recent decades, in parallel with explosive changes in clinical medicine. Advancements in such fields as neonatology, traumatology, organ transplantation and oncology have provided exciting new clinical arenas in which transfusion therapy now plays a critical role. Yet our enthusiasm for the therapeutic use of human blood has been increasingly tempered by the realization that transfusions are not necessarily benign treatment. As the clinical indications for blood transfusions have expanded, so has the list of potential transfusion hazards. It has been estimated that almost 20% of blood transfusions result in some type of adverse reaction.[1]

Hemolytic transfusion reactions are among the most feared of transfusion-associated complications, principally because acute, severe toxicity and rapid death may result. The first recorded hemolytic reactions date back to the very origin of transfusion medicine, in the mid-17th century, when animal blood was first administered to human subjects. One of the early blood recipients allegedly tolerated his first transfusion without incident, but experienced black urine, shock and death after subsequent transfusions.[2] The news of such episodes prompted the prohibition and subsequent abandonment of blood transfusion for over 150 years. It was not until Landsteiner's[3] identification of the major blood groups in 1900 that the concept of human blood compatibility was developed. Yet nearly one century later, despite a firm

Stephen M. Capon, MD, Chief, Blood Bank, Veterans Affairs Medical Center, San Diego and Dennis Goldfinger, MD, Director, Rita and Taft Schreiber Division of Transfusion Medicine, Department of Pathology and Laboratory Medicine, Cedars-Sinai Medical Center, Los Angeles, California

understanding of red cell immunology, hemolytic reactions continue to pose a constant threat to transfusion recipients. Such reactions account for over 50% of the transfusion-related fatalities in every reported series to date.[4]

Our current inability to ensure the prevention of hemolytic transfusion reactions provides ample justification for the study of this ever-timely topic. This chapter is devoted to a review of the clinical manifestations, pathophysiology and management of hemolytic transfusion reactions.

Classification and Immunology

Broadly defined, a hemolytic transfusion reaction occurs whenever the survival of red cells is shortened due to their destruction in association with a transfusion. This destruction may be immunologic and mediated by red cell antigen-antibody interactions, or it may be nonimmunologic and caused by physical or mechanical damage to transfused red cells.

Immune hemolytic transfusion reactions develop subsequent to the in-vivo interaction between a circulating antibody and its corresponding red cell antigen. In most cases, the antigen is located on the donor's erythrocytes and the antibody is found in the recipient's plasma, but reactions may also occur between donor plasma and recipient erythrocytes. The rapidity and severity of the reaction are dependent upon the characteristics of both antigen and antibody, which also determine the primary site of red cell destruction. Immune-mediated hemolytic transfusion reactions may be acute or delayed in onset, and may produce red cell lysis occurring predominantly in either the intravascular or extravascular compartments. In general, reactions characterized by intravascular hemolysis tend to be acute and more clinically devastating, whereas reactions that are manifested by extravascular hemolysis tend to be delayed and less likely to produce dangerous clinical sequelae.

When incompatible blood is transfused, red cells become sensitized, or coated with antibody. This does not, however, automatically lead to cell lysis. Certain physical properties of the antibody dictate the subsequent development and severity of hemolysis. These include 1) the antibody's immunoglobulin class (ie, IgG or IgM); 2) its ability to bind to red cells at body temperature; 3) its ability to activate the complement cascade; and 4) the presence of a binding site on the antibody for the Fc receptor of phagocytic effector cells.

The critical role of complement in the pathogenesis of hemolytic transfusion reactions has been well described.[5] Complement is activated when the C1 recognition unit contacts an antibody-bearing red cell. Initial activation requires that at least two of the five available binding sites on the C1 molecule interact with the Fc receptors of immunoglobulin on the erythrocyte surface. IgG antibody, which has only one Fc receptor per molecule, must be spaced closely enough on the red cell so that two IgG molecules can bind to a single C1 unit. Consequently, relatively high concentrations of cell-bound IgG are necessary for complement activation. In contrast, IgM antibody has a pentameric structure, and a single molecule is capable of binding to multiple C1 combining sites. Therefore, antibodies of the IgM class are more efficient at complement fixation.

After activation, the complement cascade proceeds sequentially and may terminate with C3 cleavage and inactivation, or continue to the assembly of the C5-9 membrane-attack complex. The latter forms a cylindrical macromolecule on the red cell surface that is capable of penetrating the membrane to cause immediate cell lysis. This process leads to rapid intravascular hemolysis and is responsible for the most dramatic and life-threatening transfusion reactions. Antibodies that cause immediate, complement-fixing intravascular hemolysis are usually IgM or IgG antibodies directed against ABO antigens. Most of the other naturally occurring IgM antibodies are active only at temperatures below 37 C and are rarely of clinical significance.

In some cases, red cell antibodies that fix complement are not associated with rapid intravascular hemolysis because the complement cascade is arrested after the fixation of C3. Red cells will then typically be coated with both immunoglobulins and C3d, which is an inactivated complement component. Other antibodies do not activate complement at all, but remain affixed to the erythrocyte surface. In either circumstance, sensitized red cells are not immediately hemolyzed, but are recognized and may be phagocytosed subsequently by macrophages of the reticuloendothelial system. Most clinically significant antibodies of the IgG class of immunoglobulin lead to hemolysis by one of these two mechanisms.

As a rule, red cell antibodies that activate complement cause either rapid intravascular hemolysis or extravascular hemolysis primarily within the liver. Antibodies that are unable to activate complement generally cause extravascular hemolysis within the spleen. The relationship between in-vivo and in-vitro antibody behavior is predictable but not perfect. Antibodies that are hemolytic in vitro often produce serious clinical reactions characterized by intravascular hemolysis, whereas antibodies that cause opsonization but not hemolysis in the laboratory usually cause less severe extravascular reactions.

Hemolytic transfusion reactions occasionally result from the interaction between donor-derived plasma antibodies and recipient red cells. Such "passive" hemolytic reactions are almost always caused by ABO incompatibility. Most reported cases involve the transfusion of anti-A antibody to a type A patient during the administration of whole blood, platelet concentrates or plasma components. From a clinical standpoint, this type of reaction is seldom significant. Transfused donor antibody becomes rapidly dispersed throughout the vascular compartment, yielding a state of marked antigen excess and a low concentration of bound antibody per cell. Although these conditions reduce the likelihood of hemolysis, a number of case reports describe severe, life-threatening hemolytic reactions of this type.[6,7]

An even less common type of reaction is the interdonor hemolytic transfusion reaction, which can occur in patients receiving multiple transfusions. In this circumstance, antibody introduced through the plasma of one donor reacts with incompatible red cells from another donor.[8] The resulting hemolytic reaction may vary in severity. The rarity of this reaction can be explained by the fact that screening of donor plasma for unexpected antibodies should prevent its occurrence.

Hemolytic transfusion reactions may also involve lysis of red cells in the absence of immune mechanisms. Erythrocyte survival is shortened, but the process is mediated by factors other than red cell antibodies. A temporal relationship between a blood transfusion and a hemolytic episode often exists, but may be purely coincidental. The etiologies are diverse and may be categorized by whether there is hemolysis of donor red cells, recipient red cells or both.[9]

Pathophysiology

Although the clinical features of hemolytic transfusion reactions are well known, our understanding of the specific pathophysiologic mechanisms underlying these events remains incomplete. Previous hypotheses regarding the pathogenesis of shock, disseminated intravascular coagulation (DIC) and renal failure—the three major sequelae of hemolytic reactions—have been largely conjectural in nature. However, as newer insights into the molecular basis underlying inflammation and thrombosis are gained, some revised theories of the pathogenesis of hemolytic transfusion reactions may be in order.

Traditional Concepts

Evolving beliefs regarding the mechanisms by which hemolytic transfusion reactions produce shock, DIC and renal failure have been both predicated upon and limited by the then-current understanding of inflammation and coagulation biochemical pathways. The primary initiating event has long been considered to be the release of incompatible red cell stroma-antibody complexes into the circulation. Ample experimental evidence exists to show that immune complexes are capable of activating complement, [10] platelets and the intrinsic coagulation pathway.[11-13] Complement, once activated, leads not only to the production of the C5-9 membrane-attack complex, which effectuates immediate red cell lysis, but also to the generation of several complement by-products such as C3a and C5a. These molecules serve as anaphylatoxins, which can trigger the release from mast cells of histamine and serotonin, both powerful vasodilators. Moreover, the direct activation of circulating platelets induces a secretory response leading to additional quantities of serotonin. Antigen-antibody complexes also have a stimulatory effect on Hagemen factor, leading to the activation of kallikrein and kininogen.[14] This, in turn, stimulates production of bradykinin, which also has significant vasodilatory effects.

Shock

The development of shock after a hemolytic transfusion reaction has thus been postulated as being caused by the simultaneous release of these vasoactive mediators.[14] The net effect is one of arteriolar vasodilatation, an increase in vascular permeability and a decrease in systemic blood pressure. The presence of hypotension causes the activation of compensatory regulatory mechanisms, such as the release of catecholamines by the sympathetic nervous system. This produces secondary vasoconstriction in certain vascular beds, such as the pulmonary and renal circuits, thereby creating the potential for ischemic organ injury.

The nature of the shock state produced by hemolytic transfusion reactions has generally been likened to that caused by sepsis or endotoxemia. In this setting, shock results from a "distributive" alteration in vascular volume, and is characterized by an elevated cardiac output and diminished systemic vascular resistance. This is in contrast to other types of shock, such as cardiogenic, obstructive and oligemic shock, in which very different hemodynamic derangements are observed. The presumption that shock following an incompatible transfusion is distributive in nature has been based primarily on numerous clinical similarities between severe hemolytic transfusion reactions and the sepsis syndrome, rather than on direct experimental observations.

Disseminated Intravascular Coagulation

The development of coagulation abnormalities during acute hemolytic transfusion reactions has long been a recognized phenomenon. In the 1950's and 1960's, numerous case reports were published in which patients experiencing acute hemolytic reactions developed thrombocytopenia, hypofibrinogenemia and prolongation of the prothrombin and partial thromboplastin times.[15-17] Also demonstrated was the appearance of a circulating coagulation inhibitor that was subsequently shown to represent the products of fibrin(ogen) degradation.[18] This constellation of laboratory findings is clearly consistent with DIC. During this same period, it was shown that the infusion of incompatible red cells into animals could produce both laboratory evidence of DIC and a histopathologic picture resembling the generalized Shwartzman reaction, characterized by widespread fibrin deposition within the microcirculation and multiple organ failure.[19,20]

The association between red cell hemolysis and hemostatic disturbances is not unique to hemolytic transfusion reactions. Hemolytic anemia complicated by either DIC or a thrombotic diathesis can be seen in malaria with blackwater fever, fresh water drowning, march hemoglobinuria, paroxysmal nocturnal hemoglobinuria and other conditions.[21,22]

The activation of the coagulation system to produce DIC has traditionally been considered a multifactorial process involving complement, Hageman factor and all cellular elements of the blood. Numerous mechanisms have been proposed. The release of a phospholipid substance from lysed red cells, initially termed "erythrocytin," was found to have an in-vitro procoagulant effect, and was thus postulated to be an important cause of DIC.[23] However, the infusion into animals of purified platelet factor 3, a phospholipid, has not consistently produced a coagulopathy.[24] Furthermore, the infusion of stroma-free red cell lysates was shown to have no effect on coagulation.[25] Infusions of autologous hemolysates, which contain compatible red cell membrane components, have inconsistently produced a coagulopathy,[26] whereas the administration of erythrocyte hemolysates containing incompatible stroma has produced both laboratory and pathological evidence of DIC in animal models.[27] Thus, it has been widely accepted that red cell antigen-antibody complexes in some way provide the initial stimulus to the activation of coagulation.

Immune complexes have been shown to interact independently with complement, Hageman factor, platelets and leukocytes in the laboratory setting. Numerous experimental data have linked such interactions with the activation of the intrinsic pathway of the coagulation cascade, leading to fibrin generation. The assumption that the intrinsic pathway is the primary mode of activation has been based mainly on Hageman factor consumption in experimental settings.

Acute Renal Failure

The genesis of renal failure in hemolytic transfusion reactions has been the subject of considerable debate over the years. A long-standing explanation was that the precipitation of hemoglobin within the kidney caused obstruction of the renal tubules.[28] Another hypothesis proposed that filtered free hemoglobin exerted a direct toxic effect on tubular cells.[29] These theories were largely abandoned, however, after researchers demonstrated that the infusion of stroma-free hemoglobin into animals was relatively innocuous and caused no renal dysfunction even in the setting of dehydration or acidosis.[30]

It has more recently been believed that kidney failure associated with hemolytic transfusion reactions is caused by a combination of DIC and local vasomotor changes that affect the renal microcirculation. Regardless of etiology, the development of DIC is often associated with the deposition of fibrin thrombi within the microvasculature of the kidney and acute renal failure.[31] A series of animal autopsy studies demonstrated that the renal shutdown that follows a hemolytic transfusion reaction complicated by DIC results from renal capillary thrombus formation, tubular necrosis and, in some cases, cortical infarction.[32] As described previously, systemic hypotension and secondary vasoconstriction are induced by the simultaneous generation of several vasoactive compounds. These changes lead to stasis and a reduction in renal cortical blood flow. The end result is one of renal hypoperfusion and tubular ischemia.

Several degrees of renal insufficiency may occur after an incompatible transfusion and may be viewed as resulting from variations in the severity of stasis and thrombosis within the kidney. In most cases, renal dysfunction is mild and transient. Occasionally, acute tubular necrosis occurs, which may or may not be reversible. In rare cases, bilateral renal cortical necrosis has been reported.[14,33]

The role that immune complexes have in the pathogenesis of nephrotoxicity is highlighted by the following observations. When solutions of compatible red cell stroma have been infused into humans, renal function has been unaffected, whereas infusions of incompatible stroma have resulted in acute renal failure.[34] Thus, as with production of shock and DIC, the formation of red cell stroma-antibody complexes may be ultimately responsible for the acute renal failure and, indeed, all of the adverse effects that occur after a hemolytic transfusion reaction.

Newer Concepts

During the past decade, there has been a virtual explosion of interest and knowledge regarding the molecular basis of cellular physiology. Entirely new fields of research have emerged, devoted to the study of cytokines, cellular receptors and other biochemical mediators. Out of such investigations have come exciting new insights into the mechanisms responsible for inflammation, sepsis and thrombosis. Much of this knowledge has had immediate application within the field of hematology, influencing not only our understanding of disease pathogenesis, but also the diagnosis and treatment of various hematologic disorders. In more recent years, the relevance of these concepts to transfusion medicine has begun to be explored. The pathophysiology of hemolytic transfusion reactions must be reconsidered in light of these new conceptual advancements.

Cytokines

A new class of biologic mediators, termed cytokines, has recently been discovered to be of central importance in the modulation of inflammatory and immune responses. Several of the cytokines have been cloned, recombinantly produced and studied in both laboratory and human models. Some cytokines, such as interleukin-1 (IL-1) and tumor necrosis factor (TNF), are known to have a wide range of proinflammatory and procoagulant effects and to act on many different cell types. Others, in contrast, possess more specific biologic activities and affect a limited number of target cells. The significance of these mediators in the production of human disease, although far from clarified, is now beginning to be appreciated. A number of studies have linked the production of several cytokines to the genesis of the sepsis syndrome.[35,36] Close similarities between the clinical manifestations of septic shock and those of hemolytic transfusion reactions have generated great interest in the potential roles played by cytokines in red cell incompatibility reactions.

Davenport and colleagues have constructed several in-vitro models of IgM- and IgG-mediated red cell incompatibility and studied cytokine production in experimental hemolytic transfusion reactions.[37-39] ABO incompatibility was selected as a model of IgM-mediated hemolysis, in which non-group O red cells were added to group O whole blood. IgG-mediated hemolytic reactions were studied by incubating IgG-coated red cells with mononuclear cells purified from fresh whole blood.

In the model of ABO incompatibility, several cytokines appear to be liberated in parallel with the degree of hemolysis. Following the addition of incompatible group A, but not compatible group O, red cells to group O whole blood, plasma TNF-α levels rise sharply in a dose- and time-dependent manner, peaking at 2 hours.[37] Furthermore, TNF mRNA increases measurably in mononuclear cells, indicating enhancement of TNF gene expression.

TNF is a multifunctional cytokine produced by monocytes and macrophages in response to various stimuli, especially gram-negative endotoxin. It has been demonstrated to play a pivotal role in bacterial sepsis, causing fever, hypotension and capillary leak. Thus, the release of large quantities of TNF by mononuclear cells may be an important cause of shock in acute intravascular hemolytic transfusion reactions.

In addition to TNF, interleukin-8 (IL-8) and monocyte chemoattractant protein (MCP-1) have also been detected in increased concentrations in the foregoing experiments.[39,40] IL-8 is an important chemoattractant and activator of neutrophils, while MCP-1 has similar recruiting effects on monocytes. Both are produced by monocytes, macrophages and other cell types in response to various stimuli, including IL-1, TNF and bacterial endotoxin. The generation of IL-8 and MCP-1 seems to be somewhat delayed relative to TNF, in that significant levels first appear at 4 and 6 hours, respectively, following the addition of incompatible red cells. By 24 hours, both IL-8 and MCP-1 remain in plasma, while TNF concentrations have returned to baseline.

The production and release of these cytokines may also require the presence of active complement. In the above experiments, when whole blood was replaced by washed erythrocytes and heat-treated plasma, incompatible red cells could still be agglutinated by antibody, but both hemolysis and cytokine production were abrogated.[37,39] Thus, complement could be a required intermediary for the activation of phagocytic cells in this setting.

A recent case report described the appearance of increased TNF-α in a group O patient who was accidentally transfused with 100 ml of group A red cells.[41] The patient was a participant in a study designed to investigate whether a systemic inflammatory response occurs during cardiopulmonary bypass surgery. TNF levels were found to have increased 14-fold following the incompatible transfusion and remained significantly elevated 48 hours later. In contrast, a rise in TNF levels was not observed in 19 other patients following cardiopulmonary bypass who did not receive mismatched blood. This fortuitous in-vivo observation lends weight to the in-vitro data and indicates that TNF may, indeed, be an important mediator in ABO hemolytic transfusion reactions.

Several cytokines also appear to be important in the pathogenesis of IgG-mediated hemolytic reactions. In Davenport's experimental model of IgG-mediated red cell incompatibility, IgG-sensitized erythrocytes were added to freshly isolated peripheral blood mononuclear cells.[38] Within 6 hours, the concentrations of interleukin-1 β, IL-6 and IL-8 increased significantly and remained elevated for over 24 hours. IL-1 β, like TNF, has a wide range of biologic effects including activation of neutrophils, endothelial cells and lymphocytes, and has a stimulatory effect on the production of other cytokines such as TNF, IL-6 and IL-8. IL-1 is widely believed to be a prime activator of all phases of the inflammatory response and in animal models induces fever, leukocytosis, hypotension and shock.[42] IL-6 is another important regulator of the acute phase response, and additionally has specific activity in the proliferation of T cells and the stimulation of immunoglobulin production by B cells.[43]

Unlike the above-mentioned cytokines, plasma TNF concentrations increase only transiently in IgG-mediated reactions, reaching maximal levels at 6 hours and thereafter returning to normal.[38] However, monocytes engaged in active erythrophagocytosis have been shown to express increased cell-associated TNF. The appearance of markedly elevated TNF concentrations in plasma following IgM- but not IgG-mediated hemolysis may in some way account for the clinical differences between acute and delayed type hemolytic transfusion reactions.[38]

One intriguing finding in the study of IgG-induced hemolysis has been the identification of an IL-1 receptor antagonist. Produced in monocytes in response to IgG-sensitized red cells, this protein has been detected both in culture medium suspensions as well as intracellularly in monocytes involved in the engulfment of coated erythrocytes.[44] A known inhibitor of IL-1 activity, this receptor antagonist may serve to modify or down-regulate the inflammatory response in certain hemolytic transfusion reactions.

Disseminated Intravascular Coagulation

Current concepts regarding the mechanisms of hemostasis and thrombosis have evolved rapidly and warrant a new approach to thinking about the etiology of intravascular coagulation in hemolytic transfusion reactions. A growing body of evidence now points to both leukocytes and endothelial cells as active participants in thrombogenesis and to various cytokines as critical mediators in this process. New insights have also been gained regarding the relative importance of the extrinsic pathway of coagulation activation. Formerly consigned to a comparatively minor role in thrombin generation, the Factor VII-tissue factor pathway is now considered to be the primary physiologic activator of Factor X following tissue injury.[45] The development of DIC in nearly all disease states is now believed to be triggered by the pathologic exposure, expression or release of tissue factor.

Two major cytokines, IL-1 and TNF, have been shown to play a major role in the pathogenesis of septic shock. Exaggerated production of both cytokines can be demonstrated in septic individuals as part of the inflammatory response. Animal studies have also shown that septic shock and all of its sequelae can be recreated with injections of TNF and IL-1.[46] Furthermore, passive immunization with antibodies to these cytokines prior to endotoxin challenge can block the pathological consequences and improve survival.[47]

Experimental infusions of TNF into healthy human subjects elicits the prompt and sustained activation of the common pathway of coagulation.[48] Because the contact phase of the intrinsic pathway is not activated under these conditions, it is believed that tissue factor activity is somehow increased, leading to the activation of the extrinsic pathway. In-vitro data supporting this contention include the increased synthesis and expression of thromboplastin by monocytes in response to TNF.[49] This increase in procoagulant activity appears to be caused by the increased expression of tissue factor mRNA.

Cytokines may also promote a hypercoagulable state by virtue of their effects on endothelial cells. Both IL-1 and TNF induce changes in the hemostatic properties of endothelial cell surfaces, leading to increased tissue factor and decreased thrombomodulin expression.[50,51] TNF has also been demonstrated to induce the internalization and degradation of cell-surface thrombomodulin.[52] Thrombomodulin is known to bind avidly to circulating thrombin, which in turn activates protein C zymogen. Protein C, once activated, functions as a potent anticoagulant through its proteolytic cleavage of activated Factors V and VIII. Thus, cytokine-induced down-regulation of thrombomodulin exerts a prothrombotic effect by suppression of protein C activity. Because protein C levels are decreased in sepsis-associated DIC,[53] and the infusion of purified activated protein C can prevent DIC and death in experimental models of sepsis,[54] this anticoagulant pathway is thought to be integrally involved in the pathophysiology of septic shock.

The aforementioned data have been generated during the study of DIC associated with septicemia and have not been observed directly in hemolytic transfusion reactions. However, the clinical features of severe hemolytic transfusion reactions closely resemble those of septic shock, and patterns of cytokine production are similar in both conditions. Therefore, it is likely that the mediation of intravascular coagulation occurs by similar mechanisms in both settings.

Several interesting observations have been made in experimental hemolytic transfusion reactions that shed new light on this subject. Davenport and colleagues, employing the described in-vitro model of ABO incompatibility, have demonstrated a procoagulant activity associated with peripheral blood leukocytes.[55] Following the addition of incompatible red cells to whole blood, purified lysed white cells have been shown to exert a significant procoagulant effect as measured by a one-stage, recalcified clotting time assay. This effect was not seen after the addition of ABO-compatible red cells. Activation of coagulation was shown to be due to the release of a thromboplastin-like substance acting via the extrinsic coagulation pathway. Because heat treatment abolished this procoagulant activity, complement activation may be required. The majority of this procoagulant effect was unexpectedly localized to neutrophils rather than to mononuclear cells. The precise etiology of neutrophil activation is not known, but may result from the interaction of white cell surface adhesive receptors CD11/CD18 with complement by-products localized to the surface of incompatible erythrocytes. This mechanism has been previously demonstrated to be a cause of tissue factor production in mononuclear phagocytes.[56]

As an extension of these studies, human umbilical vein endothelial cells were incubated with the plasma obtained from experimental ABO incompatibility reactions.[57] A complex response was observed, including: 1) the TNF-dependent production of IL-8 and MCP-1, chemotactic factors for neutrophils and monocytes, respectively; 2) increased gene expression for thromboplastin and for leukocyte adhesive molecules ELAM-1 and ICAM-1; and 3) the appearance of a measurable procoagulant activity. None of these findings was observed using plasma from ABO-compatible reactions. These exciting observations are consistent with the growing realization that endothelial cells are active participants in both inflammation and thrombosis.

Renal Failure

The mechanisms of renal injury in hemolytic transfusion reactions have been largely speculative, as discussed above. However, recent advances in vascular endothelial physiology and research in the field of artificial blood substitutes have provided new clues to the understanding of renal dysfunction.

In recent years, it has been recognized that endothelial cells produce a variety of vasoactive mediators that regulate vascular smooth muscle tone in response to different stimuli.[58] Of these, endothelium-derived relaxing factor and endothelin appear to be biologically significant. Endothelium-derived relaxing factor has been identified to be at least in part nitric oxide.[59] Derived from intracellular L-arginine, nitric oxide causes a decrease in vascular smooth muscle tone to produce a vasodilatory effect. In contrast, endothelin is a powerful vasoconstrictor and is currently the most potent endogenous vasoactive substance identified in humans.[60] Within the kidney, vascular resistance, and thus renal perfusion, appears to be controlled to a large degree by a balance between these vasodilatory and vasoconstricting factors.[61]

The release of endothelin from vascular tissue has been shown to be induced by thrombin, bradykinin, epinephrine and IL-1.[62] It may be hypothesized that following a hemolytic transfusion reaction, the exposure of renal endothelium to these substances may produce endothelin release and subsequent local vasoconstriction, leading to parenchymal ischemia and possibly acute renal failure.

New insights into endothelial physiology may also provide clues to the long-debated question of direct hemoglobin nephrotoxicity. It has been recognized for years that hemoglobinemia is associated with significant vasomotor effects. From the earliest work on red blood cell substitutes, the administration of hemoglobin-saline solutions to both animals and humans produced hypertension on a frequent basis.[63] In a recent study in which acutely bled swine were resuscitated with various fluids, the infusion of native or cross-linked hemoglobin caused increases in systemic vascular resistance that were greater than twice that observed when equal volumes of crystalloid or colloid solutions were used.[64] In the hemoglobin-treated animals, marked elevations in blood pressure were associated with significant and even fatal reductions in cardiac output. The hemodynamic changes appeared to result from severe generalized vasoconstriction.

A potential explanation for this apparent hemoglobin-induced vasoconstrictive effect may relate to its interaction with nitric oxide. Cell-free hemoglobin has been shown to tightly bind nitric oxide via attachment to the heme moiety, and in doing so may eliminate its biologic transduction properties.[65] It is now believed that circulating hemoglobin, perhaps following egress into subendothelial tissues, binds nitric oxide, inhibits its vasorelaxant properties and causes localized vasoconstriction. This has been suggested to be the etiology of hypertension, chest pain and several other signs and symptoms observed in volunteer recipients of a variety of investigational hemoglobin solutions. While clearly posing a roadblock to the development of artificial blood substitutes, these observations may also shed new light on the genesis of tissue injury in acute hemolytic transfusion reactions. The liberation of large quantities of free hemoglobin may, by this mechanism, alter vascular smooth muscle tone to produce vasoconstriction and consequent organ ischemia. This may be particularly relevant to the pathogenesis of acute renal failure, given the sensitivity of the kidney to vasomotor disturbances within the renal microcirculation.

A particularly interesting discovery has been that inhibition of endothelial-derived nitric oxide can lead to enhanced leukocyte adhesion to endothelium and subsequent invasion of vessel walls.[66] Thus, the presence of hemoglobin in the circulation may, by this mechanism, lead to localized inflammation in a variety of tissues. The relevance of this finding to renal disease is entirely unknown. Thus far, leukocyte-derived cytokines have not been found to be directly involved in the pathogenesis of acute renal failure in any clinical setting.

Clearly, the etiology of acute renal failure in hemolytic transfusion reactions appears to be a complex and multifactorial process. In severe reactions accompanied by shock and DIC, renal hypoperfusion and widespread fibrin deposition are still likely to be key factors in renal ischemia. The newer theories put forth suggest that endothelial-derived autocoids, in part influenced by free hemoglobin, may play an important additive role.

Acute Respiratory Failure

The lungs have not traditionally been regarded as a target organ in hemolytic transfusion reactions. However, acute impairment of pulmonary function can accompany the state of multiorgan failure that may develop in the most severe cases. In some patients experiencing acute hemolytic transfusion reactions who have been monitored in the ICU setting, hypoxemic and/or hypercapneic respiratory failure has been occasionally observed. In severe cases, profound respiratory failure has developed, characterized by pulmonary edema or an adult respiratory distress syndrome (ARDS)-like picture.

An interesting case report recently described the hemodynamic changes that occurred in a patient who accidentally received ABO incompatible blood while being aggressively monitored.[67] Immediately after the transfusion began, an increase in pulmonary vascular resistance and pulmonary artery pressure developed, accompanied by a decrease in stroke volume and cardiac output. Blood pressure was maintained by reflex tachycardia. The transfusion was halted before any further complications developed, and all hemodynamic parameters returned to baseline. This pattern of initial response appeared to be consistent with acute obstruction in the pulmonary vascular circuit.

The pathophysiologic mechanisms underlying these changes are not well understood, but several hypotheses may be considered. Upon entry of incompatible blood into the circulation, complement-mediated red cell lysis occurs, resulting in hemoglobinemia. As the quantity of liberated hemoglobin starts to exceed haptoglobin binding capacity, free plasma hemoglobin accumulates. The passage of free hemoglobin through the pulmonary vascular bed may interact with endothelial-derived nitric oxide, leading to localized vasoconstriction. As the process evolves further, pulmonary vascular hypertension and decreased cardiac output may then develop.

TNF has been implicated in the development of septic ARDS, in part related to its effect on neutrophil stimulation, adhesion and superoxide production.[68] The release of TNF during acute hemolytic reactions may, by similar mechanisms, participate in acute lung injury. The enzyme neutrophil elastase has been observed to increase markedly in plasma following an incompatible transfusion.[41] The release of large quantities of this enzyme via neutrophil degranulation has been suggested to be partly responsible for the pulmonary capillary endothelial injury that occurs in ARDS and could also be an important cause of pulmonary compromise in acute hemolytic transfusion reactions. Additional tissue injury may occur if pulmonary endothelial cells express leukocyte adhesion molecules, liberate neutrophil and monocyte chemotactic factors such as IL-8 and MCP-1 or generate a local procoagulant activity, all of which promote localized inflammation and thrombosis.

Thus, acute respiratory failure should be anticipated as a possible consequence of severe hemolytic transfusion reactions. Furthermore, the development of hypoxemia and acidosis arising from acute lung injury undoubtedly contributes to systemic hemodynamic changes and distant organ ischemia.

Treatment Considerations

Two important principles continue to guide the management of hemolytic transfusion reactions. First, the clinical severity of any hemolytic reaction is directly proportional to the volume of incompatible blood transfused. Therefore, as soon as a hemolytic reaction is suspected, the transfusion must be promptly stopped. Second, the life-threatening sequelae of hemolytic transfusion reactions can be favorably influenced and potentially prevented by early therapeutic intervention. When such a reaction is judged to be present, emergency treatment must precede definitive establishment of the diagnosis. While awaiting laboratory confirmation of a hemolytic reaction, the traditional approach to patient management has included the establishment of large vessel venous access, careful monitoring of vital signs and the administration of diuretics to enhance urine output.

In view of what is now known about the pathophysiology of hemolytic transfusion reactions, a somewhat more aggressive course of action can be recommended. As soon as a transfusion recipient exhibits clinical evidence of a true hemolytic reaction, such as unstable vital signs, persistent chest pain or respiratory distress, the patient should be transferred to an intensive care unit (ICU) for closer observation. If a clerical check reveals that an ABO-incompatible transfusion has been inadvertently given, one may anticipate the possibility of a clinically severe course. In this circumstance, ICU transfer should be entertained regardless of the patient's immediate status. The placement of a Swan-Ganz catheter should be considered at the first sign of hemodynamic instability and perhaps in all recipients of a significant volume of ABO-incompatible red cells. Right heart catheterization is a relatively low risk procedure that permits precise measurement of pulmonary arterial pressures, cardiac output and left atrial filling pressures, and allows rapid calculation of systemic and pulmonary vascular resistances. Such information can be an invaluable guide to the administration of fluids in the hypotensive or oliguric patient, the selection and monitoring of vasopressor agents for treatment of shock, and the judicious use of vasodilators to address heart failure caused by pulmonary or systemic hypertension. Without the benefit of such invasive monitoring, clinicians are forced to utilize an unacceptable degree of guesswork and empiricism in the management of a potentially fatal illness.

The choice of an optimal diuretic agent has been the subject of considerable historical debate. Both mannitol and loop diuretics, such as furosemide, have been utilized to enhance urinary output and prevent acute renal failure following an incompatible transfusion. Both drugs effectively enhance renal blood flow and diuresis, yet each has unique disadvantages. Mannitol, being a powerful osmotic agent, can cause a sudden transient increase in intravascular volume and blood pressure, leading to pulmonary edema. Furosemide, in contrast, has the potential of inducing an undesirable hypotensive response. The proper selection of a diuretic should be based on the patient's hemodynamic and fluid status at the time. Mannitol would be preferable if hypotension or shock has developed, whereas a loop diuretic would be the better choice if there are signs of fluid overload or hypertension.

The treatment of hypotension is also made simpler and more effective with invasive hemodynamic monitoring. Aggressive fluid replacement with crystalloid solutions can usually be continued safely until left atrial filling pressures are optimized; thereafter, infusion of vasopressor agents may be considered. Dopamine should be the initial pressor of choice because it has a vasodilatory effect on renal vascular beds when used in relatively low doses. In view of this potentially protective effect on kidney function, an infusion of dopamine (1-5 µg/kg/min) should be considered even in the absence of a need for blood pressure support.

The management of DIC has traditionally included the cautious administration of red cells, platelet concentrates and plasma components as replacement therapy in the bleeding patient. The use of heparin in all forms of DIC has long been considered controversial, but may be indicated where a thrombotic diathesis complicates the coagulopathy. Several studies have shown that most serious hemolytic transfusion reactions take place in surgical operating rooms and intensive care units,[69,70] settings in which full-dose anticoagulation may be hazardous. Nonetheless, the early institution of heparin has been recommended in selected patients in order to slow the consumptive process.[14,71] When used, a standard loading dose of 5000 units should be followed by the infusion of 1000 to 1500 units per hour. Close monitoring of the patient's coagulation parameters is thereafter essential.

Respiratory distress can be managed with oxygen administration and, if necessary, mechanical ventilation. The institution of early intubation and ventilatory support is preferable to postponing such action until a prolonged period of hypoxemia has elapsed.

Future Treatment Strategies

At the present time, management principles are based primarily on supportive treatment of the known complications of hemolytic transfusion reactions. However, in light of our growing understanding of the pathogenesis of these events, future therapeutic interventions are likely to be aimed at modulation of the underlying pathophysiologic mechanisms. The goals of such intervention will be the down-regulation of the immune response and the inhibition of coagulation pathways.

Given the now-recognized prominent role that cytokines play in the mediation of infection and the systemic inflammatory response, much work is being done to determine whether inhibition of these cytokines can ameliorate the course of various disease states. Experimental strategies for reducing the effects of cytokines may be nonspecific or specific in nature. For example, corticosteroids have been found to nonspecifically inhibit transcriptional and posttranscriptional expression of IL-1 in cell culture.[72] Specific blockade of IL-1 and TNF is now possible by a variety of methods and, in both animal models and early clinical trials in humans, appears to hold promise in the treatment of systemic inflammatory conditions.[73] TNF antagonism can be accomplished through the administration of monoclonal antibodies to TNF or soluble TNF receptors. Both are capable of neutralizing circulating TNF and appear to be efficacious in reducing the severity of inflammation and improving survival in bacteremic shock states.[74,75] Inhibition of IL-1 can be accomplished by the administration of IL-1 receptor antagonist,[76] antibodies to IL-1 receptors[77] or soluble IL-1 receptors.[78] Several of these agents are currently in Phase II or III trials in the treatment of sepsis.[73]

On the basis of their known immunomodulatory actions, several of these agents may prove to be of value in the treatment of hemolytic transfusion reactions. It can be postulated that the maximal benefit of these therapies will require their introduction early in the course of hemolytic reactions in order to be effective. It may eventually be shown that a multimodality approach involving the specific blockade of IL-1 and TNF, as well as nonspecific immune modulation, will be necessary in order to achieve a clinical benefit. The future utilization of this type of therapy will obviously require the completion of Phase III trials now in progress, as well as preliminary laboratory and animal studies utilizing experimental models of hemolytic transfusion reactions.

New advances in coagulation research may soon yield novel and clinically useful inhibitors of thrombin generation. It is now known that the extrinsic coagulation pathway, initiated by Factor VII-tissue factor interaction, is of far greater physiologic importance than previously appreciated.[45] Tissue factor is generally believed to be responsible for triggering DIC in gram-negative endotoxemia, malignant neoplasms and, possibly, hemolytic transfusion reactions. The primary physiologic inhibitor of this pathway has been identified as tissue factor pathway inhibitor (TFPI), which can now be measured and correlated with various states of coagulation activation.[79] The development of a purified and clinically safe form of TFPI may one day herald a new era in anticoagulation therapy. Among its many potential clinical uses may be the treatment of DIC in hemolytic transfusion reactions.

An equally exciting prospect is the development of purified protein C concentrates. The activated form of protein C, one of two vitamin K-dependent natural anticoagulants, catalyzes the proteolytic cleavage of Factors Va and VIIIa, thereby abrogating their coagulation cofactor function. Ongoing research may reveal that protein C concentrates provide yet another tool in the treatment of thrombotic disorders.

The clinical investigation of hemolytic transfusion reactions provides a fascinating window into the study of human physiology and immunology. Clearly, much remains to be learned. As knowledge is gained about the mechanisms that govern the course of hemolytic transfusion reactions, the prospects for better therapy and improved survival appear ever brighter.

Acknowledgment

The authors thank Dianne Johnson for expert assistance in manuscript preparation and editing.

References

1. Walker RH. Special report: Transfusion risks. Am J Clin Pathol 1987;88:374-8.
2. Weiner AS. Blood groups and transfusion. Springfield, IL: Thomas, 1943:50-9.
3. Landsteiner K. Zur Kenntnis der antifermentativen, lytischen und agglutinierenden Wirkungen des Blutserums und des Lymphe. Zentralbl Bakteriol Mikrobiol Hyg 1900;27:357-62.
4. Myrhe BA. Fatalities from blood transfusion. JAMA 1980;244:1333-5.
5. Garratty G. The significance of complement in immunohematology. CRC Crit Rev Clin Lab Sci 1984;20:25-56.
6. Zoes C, Dube VE, Miller HJ, Vye MV. Anti A$_1$ in the plasma of platelet concentrates causing a hemolytic reaction. Transfusion 1977;17:29-32.
7. Conway LT, Scott EP. Acute hemolytic transfusion reaction due to ABO incompatible plasma in a plateletpheresis concentrate. Transfusion 1989;24:413-4.
8. West NC, Jenkins JA, Johnston BR, Modi N. Interdonor incompatibility due to anti-Kell antibody undetected by automated antibody screening. Vox Sang 1986;50:174-6.

9. Capon SM, Sacher RA. Hemolytic transfusion reactions: A review of mechanisms, sequelae, and management. J Intensive Care Med 1989;4:100-11.
10. Ruddy S, Gigli I, Austen KF. The complement system in man. N Engl J Med 1972;287:489-95.
11. Pfueller SL, Luscher EF. Studies of the mechanisms of the human platelet release reaction induced by immunologic stimuli. I. Complement-dependent and complement-independent reactions. J Immunol 1974;112:201-8.
12. Kaplan AP, Gigli I, Austen KF. Immunologic activation of Hageman factor and its relationship to fibrinolysis, bradykinin generation and complement. J Clin Invest 1971;50:51a.
13. Ratnoff OD. Some relationships among hemostasis, fibrinolytic phenomena, immunity, and the inflammatory response. Adv Immunol 1969;10:145-50.
14. Goldfinger D. Acute hemolytic transfusion reactions—a fresh look at pathogenesis and considerations regarding therapy. Transfusion 1977;17:85-98.
15. Krevans JR, Jackson DP, Conley CL, Hartmann RC. The nature of the hemorrhagic disorder accompanying hemolytic transfusion reactions in man. Blood 1957;12:834-43.
16. Moore JM. Uncontrollable post-operative haemorrhage after incompatible blood transfusion. Br Med J 1958;2:1201-3.
17. Ingram GIC. The bleeding complications of blood transfusion. Transfusion 1965;5:1-5.
18. Sack ES, Nefa OM. Fibrinogen and fibrin degradation products in hemolytic transfusion reactions. Transfusion 1970;10:317-21.
19. McKay DG, Hardaway RM, Wahle GH, et al. Alterations in blood coagulation mechanisms after incompatible blood transfusion. Am J Surg 1955;89:583-92.
20. Hardaway RM, McKay DG, Wahle GH, et al. Pathologic study of intravascular coagulation following incompatible blood transfusion in dogs. I. Intravenous injection of incompatible blood. Am J Surg 1956;91:24-31.
21. Newcomb TF, Gardner FH. Thrombin generation in paroxysmal nocturnal hemoglobinuria. Br J Haematol 1963;9:84-90.
22. Reidler G, Frick PG, Straub PW. The effects of intravascular hemolysis on coagulation and fibrinolysis. II. March hemoglobinemia and hemoglobinuria. Helvetica Med Acta 1968;34:217-22.
23. Hussey CV, Kaser MM. Erythrocytin, a clotting factor from erythrocytes: Its action and purification. Fed Proc 1956;15:279-82.
24. Goldfinger D. Intravenous infusion of partial thromboplastin in rabbits. Fed Proc 1966;25:255.
25. Rabiner SF, Helbert JR, Lopas H, Friedman LH. Evaluation of stroma-free hemoglobin solution for use as a plasma expander. J Exp Med 1967;126:1127-42.

26. Rabiner SF, Friedman LH. The role of intravascular hemolysis and the reticuloendothelial system in the production of hypercoagulable state. Br J Haematol 1968;14:105-18.

27. Birndorf NI, Lopas H. Intravascular coagulation in cynomolgus monkeys produced by red cell stroma (abstract). Clin Res 1970;18:398.

28. Baker SL, Dodds EC. Obstruction of the renal tubules during the excretion of haemoglobin. Br J Exp Pathol 1925;6:247.

29. Bing RJ. The effect of hemoglobin and related pigments on renal functions of the normal and acidotic dog. Bull Johns Hopkins Hospital 1944;74:161-76.

30. Relihan M, Olsen RE, Litwin MS. Clearance rate and effect on renal function of stroma-free hemoglobin following renal ischemia. Ann Surg 1972;176:700-4.

31. Regoeczi E, Brain MC. Organ distribution of fibrin in disseminated intravascular coagulation. Br J Haematol 1969;17:73-81.

32. Hardaway RM, McKay DG. Changes in the dog kidney produced by incompatible blood transfusion. Arch Surg 1959;78:565-73.

33. Muirhead EE. Incompatible blood transfusions with emphasis on acute renal failure. Surg Gynecol Obstet 1951;92:734-46.

34. Schmidt PJ, Holland PV. Pathogenesis of the acute renal failure associated with incompatible transfusion. Lancet 1967;2:1169-72.

35. Billiau A, Vandekerckhove F. Cytokines and their interactions with other inflammatory mediators in the pathogenesis of sepsis and septic shock. Eur J Clin Invest 1991;21:559-73.

36. Cannon JG, Tompkins RG, Gelfand FA, et al. Circulating interleukin-1 and tumor necrosis factor in septic shock and experimental endotoxin fever. J Infect Dis 1990;161:79-84.

37. Davenport RD, Streiter RM, Kunkel SL. Red cell ABO incompatibility and production of tumour necrosis factor-alpha. Br J Haematol 1991;78:540-4.

38. Davenport RD, Burdick M, Moore SA, Kunkel SL. Cytokine production in IgG-mediated red cell incompatibility. Transfusion 1993;33:19-24.

39. Davenport RD, Streiter RM, Standiford TJ, Kunkel SL. Interleukin-8 production in red blood cell incompatibility. Blood 1990;76:2439-42.

40. Davenport RD, Burdick M, Streiter RM, Kunkel SL. Monocyte chemoattractant protein production in red cell incompatibility. Transfusion 1993 (in press).

41. Butler J, Parker D, Pillai R, et al. Systemic release of neutrophil elastase and tumour necrosis factor alpha following ABO incompatible blood transfusion. Br J Haematol 1991;79:525-6.

42. Dinarello CA. Interleukin-1 and interleukin-1 antagonism. Blood 1991;77:1627-52.

43. Le J, Vilcek J. Interleukin 6: A multifunctional cytokine regulating immune reactions and the acute phase protein response. Lab Invest 1989;61:588-602.

44. Davenport RD, Burdick M, Streiter RM, Kunkel SL. Interleukin-1 receptor antagonist (IL-1ra) production in IgG mediated hemolysis (abstract). Transfusion 1992;32(Suppl):45S.
45. Rappaport SI. Blood coagulation and its alterations in hemorrhagic and thrombotic disorders. West J Med 1993;158:153-61.
46. Tracey KJ, Beutler B, Lowry SF, et al. Shock and tissue injury induced by human recombinant cachectin. Science 1986;234:470-4.
47. Beveler B, Milsark IW, Cerami AC. Passive immunization against cachectin/tumor necrosis factor protects mice from lethal effect of endotoxin. Science 1985;229:869-71.
48. Van der Poll T, Buller HR, Ten Cate H, et al. Activation of coagulation after administration of tumor necrosis factor to normal subjects. N Engl J Med 1990;322:1622-7.
49. Conkling PR, Greenberg CS, Weinberg JB. Tumor necrosis factor induces tissue factor-like activity in human leukemia cell line U937 and peripheral blood monocytes. Blood 1988;72:128-33.
50. Nawroth PP, Handley DA, Esmon CT, Stern DM. Interleukin-1 induces endothelial cell procoagulant while suppressing cell surface anticoagulant activity. Proc Natl Acad Sci USA 1986;83:3460-4.
51. Nawroth PP, Stern DM. Modulation of endothelial cell hemostatic properties by tumor necrosis factor. J Exp Med 1986;163:740-4.
52. Moore KL, Esmon CT, Esmon NL. Tumor necrosis factor leads to the internalization and degradation of thrombomodulin from the surface of bovine aortic endothelial cells in culture. Blood 1989; 73:159-65.
53. Griffin JH, Mosher DF, Zimmerman TS, Kleiss AJ. Protein C, an antithrombotic protein, is reduced in hospitalized patients with intravascular coagulation. Blood 1982;60:261-5.
54. Taylor FB, Chang A, Esmon CT, et al. Protein C prevents the coagulopathic and lethal effects of *E. coli* infusion in the baboon. J Clin Invest 1987;79:918-21.
55. Davenport RD, Kunkel SL. Leukocyte procoagulant activity induced by ABO incompatibility. Blood 1993 (in press).
56. Fan S-T, Edgington TS. Coupling of the adhesive receptor CDllb/CD18 to functional enhancement of effector macrophage tissue factor response. J Clin Invest 1991;87:50-6.
57. Davenport RD, Burdick M, Kunkel SL. Endothelial cell activation in hemolytic transfusion reactions (abstract). Transfusion 1992; 32(Suppl):53S.
58. Brenner BM, Troy JL, Ballermann BJ. Endothelium-dependent vascular responses. J Clin Invest 1989;84:1373-8.
59. Palmer RMJ, Ashton DS, Moncada S. Vascular endothelial cells synthesize nitric oxide from L-arginine. Nature (Lond) 1988;333: 664-6.

60. Yanagisawa M, Kurihara H, Kimura S, et al. A novel potent vasoconstrictor peptide produced by vascular endothelial cells. Nature (Lond) 1988;332:411-5.
61. Griendling KK, Lassegue BP, Taylor WR, Alexander RW. Control of vascular tone by the endothelium: New insights. J Crit Illness 1993;8:355-70.
62. Kon V, Badr KF. Biological actions and pathophysiologic significance of endothelin in the kidney. Kidney Int 1991;40:1-12.
63. Amberson WR, Jennings JJ, Rhode CM. Clinical experience with hemoglobin-saline solutions. J Appl Physiol 1949;1:469-89.
64. Hess JR, MacDonald VW, Brinkley WW. Systemic and pulmonary hypertension after resuscitation with cell-free hemoglobin. J Appl Physiol 1993 (in press).
65. Moncada SR, Palmer MJ, Higgs EA. Nitric oxide: Physiology, pathophysiology, and pharmacology. Pharmacol Rev 1991;40: 109-42.
66. Kubes P, Suzuki M, Granger DN. Nitric oxide: An endogenous modulator of leukocyte adhesion. Proc Natl Acad Sci USA 1991; 88:4651-5.
67. Goldfinger D, O'Connell M, Ellrodt AG. Pathogenesis and treatment of shock associated with acute hemolytic transfusion reactions (abstract). Transfusion 1985;25:468.
68. Tracey KJ, Lowry SF, Cerami A. Cachectin/TNF in septic shock and septic adult respiratory distress syndrome. Am Rev Respir Dis 1988;137:1377-9.
69. Schmidt PJ. Transfusion mortality, with special reference to surgical and intensive care facilities. J Fla Med Assoc 1980;67:151-6.
70. Honig CL, Bove JR. Transfusion associated fatalities: Review of Bureau of Biologics reports. Transfusion 1980;20:653-61.
71. Rock RC, Bove JR, Nemerson Y. Heparin treatment of intravascular coagulation accompanying hemolytic transfusion reactions. Transfusion 1969;9:57-61.
72. Knudsen PJ, Dinarello CA, Strom TB. Glucocorticoids inhibit transcriptional and posttranscriptional expression of interleukin 1 in U937 cells. J Immunol 1987;139:4129-34.
73. Dinarello CA, Gelfand JA, Wolff SM. Anticytokine strategies in the treatment of the systemic inflammatory response syndrome. JAMA 1993;269:1829-35.
74. Tracey K, Fong Y, Hesse DG, et al. Anti-cachectin/TNF monoclonal antibodies prevent septic shock during lethal bacteremia. Nature 1987;330:662-4.
75. van Zee KJ, Kohno T, Fischer E, et al. Tumor necrosis factor soluble receptors circulate during experimental and clinical inflammation and can protect against excessive tumor necrosis factor-α in vitro and in vivo. Proc Natl Acad Sci USA 1992;89: 4845-9.

76. Arend WP. Interleukin 1 receptor antagonist: A new member of the interleukin family. J Clin Invest 1991;88:1445-51.
77. Gershenwald JE, Fong YM, Fahey TJ III, et al. Interleukin 1 receptor blockage attenuates the host inflammatory response. Proc Natl Acad Sci USA 1990;87:4966-70.
78. Fanslow WC, Sims JE, Sassenfeld H, et al. Regulation of alloreactivity in vivo by a soluble form of the interleukin-1 receptor. Science 1990;248:739-42.
79. Warr TA, Rao LVM, Rappaport SI. Human plasma extrinsic pathway inhibitor activity. II. Plasma levels in disseminated intravascular coagulation and hepatocellular disease. Blood 1989;74:994-8.

In: Nance ST, ed.
Alloimmunity: 1993 and Beyond
Bethesda, MD: American Association of Blood Banks, 1993

7

Prenatal and Perinatal Management of Alloimmune Cytopenias

Janice G. McFarland, MD

ONGENITAL ANEMIA, THROMBOCYTOPENIA, and neutropenia can all be associated with maternal alloantibodies specific for antigens on erythrocytes, platelets and neutrophils, respectively. The focus of this chapter will be on the clinical management of hemolytic disease of the newborn (and fetus) (HDN) due to non-ABO antigens and neonatal (and fetal) alloimmune thrombocytopenia purpura (NATP). Neonatal alloimmune neutropenia will not be addressed.

HDN: Overview

Hydrops fetalis and kernicterus were described in detail around the turn of the century, but were not considered to be related until 1932, when Diamond et al showed that these two conditions together with icterus gravis were different manifestations of the same disease.[1] Other features of the disease included hemolytic anemia, extramedullary erythropoiesis, hepatosplenomegaly and nucleated red cells in the peripheral blood—hence the term "erythroblastosis fetalis."

In 1939, Levine and Stetson suggested that the condition was related to maternal sensitization to a paternal red cell antigen. They described a woman who had a severe transfusion reaction to her husband's blood after delivering a hydropic stillborn infant.[2] In 1940, the identity of the offending antigen was found after Landsteiner and Weiner's experiments involving immunization of guinea pigs and rabbits with rhesus monkey red cells. The red cell antibodies produced reacted with 85% of red cell samples from Caucasians.[3] Levine quickly

Janice G. McFarland, MD, Acting Medical Director, The Blood Center of Southeastern Wisconsin, Milwaukee, Wisconsin

demonstrated that his patient's red cells were Rh-negative while those of her husband were Rh positive. Moreover, she was found to have an antibody that agglutinated her husband's red cells and the red cells of other Rh-positive individuals but not those of Rh-negative people.[4]

Pathophysiology

By the early 1940's, the etiology of HDN was established. A woman lacking a particular red cell antigen, after exposure to blood positive for the antigen, makes antibodies reactive with the antigen. The IgG red cell antibody crosses the placenta into the fetal circulation and coats the fetal incompatible red cells, causing their destruction. This ongoing destruction of fetal red cells with its consequent anemia and hyperbilirubinemia accounts for the clinical features of HDN: severe anemia with high output cardiac failure (hydrops), hepatomegaly with portal hypertension, hyperbilirubinemia and kernicterus (toxic accumulation of indirect bilirubin in the brain). Although the Rh antigen (D) historically accounted for the bulk of HDN cases, other red cell alloantigens are capable of immunizing pregnant women, resulting in the disease (Table 7-1).

We now recognize that the major source of exposure of Rh-negative women to Rh-positive blood occurs in pregnancy. The most severely affected cases of HDN occurred in multiparous women who had had unaffected or only mildly affected children in the past. The fetal transplacental hemorrhage theory held that during a first pregnancy with an incompatible fetus, a small number of fetal red cells enter the maternal circulation at delivery. These then cause primary immunization of the mother who, during subsequent pregnancies, has anamnes-

Table 7-1. Red Cell Antibodies Associated With Moderate or Severe HDN

System	Specificities
Rh	Anti-D,-c, -C, C^w, -C^x, -e, -E, -E^w, -ce, -Ce^s, -Rh32, -Go^a, -Be^a, -Evans, -Riv, -LW
Kell	Anti-K, -Js^a, -Js^b, -Ku
Kidd	Anti-Jk^a
Duffy	Anti-Fy^a
MNSs	Anti-M, -N, -s, -U
Other	Anti-PP_1P^k, -Di^b, -Lan, -LW, -Far, -Good, -Wr^a, -Zd

(Modified from Mollison et al.[5])

tic recall of the anti-red cell immune response, resulting in progressively more severely affected fetuses.

The theory was supported by a case reported by Chown,[6] in which an Rh-negative woman gave birth to a severely anemic neonate without serologic evidence of anti-D. The mother was shown to have a large amount (8%) of circulating fetal cells. About three weeks later, she developed anti-D and subsequent pregnancies were severely affected with HDN.

The development of the acid elution test of Kleihauer et al in 1957[7] allowed more precise quantitation of fetomaternal transplacental hemorrhage (FMH). Transplacental hemorrhage is, in fact, very common during pregnancy and immediately after delivery and can be detected in up to 76% of pregnancies when monitoring is done throughout gestation and shortly after delivery. The majority of FMHs take place in the third trimester and after delivery.[8]

Clinical Features

Rh disease can be associated with severe fetal anemia and the development of hydrops fetalis and in-utero death as early as 20-24 weeks of gestation.[9] Hydrops fetalis, in its fullest extent, includes anemia, hepatosplenomegaly, ascites and edema associated with high output heart failure.

The amount of maternal antibody (IgG) transported across the placenta is known to increase as gestation progresses, becoming maximal late in the third trimester.[10] Therefore, it is unusual to detect significant anemia before 20 weeks of gestation. However, once anemia develops, it worsens with advanced gestation dependent on increased maternal antibody entering the fetal circulation. The inefficient transport of maternal antibody to the fetus earlier in pregnancy probably explains why even very severely affected fetuses will not develop hydrops prior to 20 weeks. Hydrops itself requires an extremely severe degree of fetal anemia to manifest, and some fetuses have hematocrits less than 0.10 (10%) before hydrops occurs.[11]

Therefore, fetal hydrops only occurs when severe anemia is present, but severe anemia may be present without the development of fetal hydrops.

Antenatal Management of HDN

With the demonstration by the 1940's that exchange transfusions successfully salvaged about one-half of the liveborn infants with severe HDN,[12] attention turned to antenatal therapy to reduce the incidence of severely affected hydropic fetuses. Several important tools help in predicting affected fetuses and the severity of HDN.

Maternal History—Prior Pregnancy Outcomes

In general, the severity of HDN remains the same or increases in subsequent affected pregnancies. If a mother presents with a history of delivering hydropic fetuses in the past, a subsequent affected fetus can be expected to have a greater than 90% chance of being similarly affected.[12] This complication will usually occur at about the same gestational age or before that in the previous pregnancy. In a first sensitized pregnancy, no maternal history is available with which to predict disease severity. In this situation, the overall risk of having a hydropic fetus is 8-10%.[12]

Using the severity of prior affected pregnancies to predict the outcome of a current pregnancy is complicated in the case of a father who is heterozygous for the implicated antigen. If such information is available, attempts to ascertain the fetal blood type may be justified before monitoring the pregnancy for the development of hemolysis and hydrops. Early fetal blood type determination using chorionic villus samples from fetuses as early as 8 weeks of gestation has been reported.[13-15] Later in gestation, at 18-20 weeks, fetal blood can be obtained for typing. The risk of further immunizing the mother by procedures to determine fetal blood type must be considered. It is estimated that percutaneous umbilical blood sampling (PUBS) may increase the subsequent degree of alloimmunization by about 50%.[16] Therefore, Rh immune globulin (RhIG) prophylaxis is indicated after such procedures.

If the fetus is found to have the incompatible blood type, prospective monitoring for disease severity can proceed as described below, depending on the maternal history. If, however, the fetus is found to not have the offending antigen, monitoring for HDN is not necessary.

Maternal Alloantibody Titers

Antibody titrations performed in the same laboratory in a consistent manner can provide some indication of risk that a particular pregnancy will be complicated by severe HDN. They are not, however, accurate enough to be the sole tool for deciding when antenatal intervention should be undertaken. Bowman and Pollock estimate that the accuracy of severity predictions made on the basis of antibody titers is only about 62%.[17]

In general, an anti-D titer of 1:16 or a significant elevation of titer in an immunized pregnant mother are indications for amniocentesis after 20 weeks of gestation.[18] Mollison contends that estimations of maternal antibody concentration in the Autoanalyzer are better correlated with severity of HDN than are antibody titers.[5] In one series of 78 alloimmunized mothers, whose anti-D concentration remained less than 4 IU/mL (0.8 μg/mL), no infant had a cord hemoglobin level less than 100 g/L (10g/dL) and only three needed exchange transfusions. In contrast, among 106 mothers with anti-D levels greater than 4 IU/mL, 23 infants had cord hemoglobin concentrations less than 100 g/L (10 g/dL) and 79 required exchange transfusion.[19]

The AABB recommends screening for unexpected antibodies in the first trimester and again at 28 weeks of gestation if the woman is Rh-negative to confirm lack of anti-D and, therefore, appropriateness of the 28-week dose of RhIG.[18] Rh-positive women who have no unexpected antibodies detected in the initial first-trimester screen need not have a repeat screening done later in pregnancy. Those women who have anti-D detected in the first-trimester screen should undergo repeat antibody titration every 2-4 weeks after 20 weeks of gestation. Women with anti-D titers at or in excess of 1:16 should undergo amniocentesis to assess the severity of HDN (see below). Repeat testing for titration of non-anti-D antibodies should be considered if the initial first-trimester screen revealed unexpected antibodies or if there is a previous history of such antibodies being detected. No critical titer has been established for non-anti-D antibodies, and rarely is antenatal intervention warranted for these cases.[18]

Innovative methods of measuring anti-D using monocyte phagocytosis of antibody-coated red cells[20] or antibody-dependent cell-mediated cytotoxicity (ADCC)[21,22] have been reported to be even more accurate in predicting the severity of HDN than the standard indirect antiglobulin method.

The presence and titer of anti-D in the maternal circulation are easily measured and are useful indicators of active disease if there is a significant increase in the titer. However, the titer of alloantibody by itself is not very specific and does not distinguish mildly affected from severely affected cases. In addition, several cases are known in which previously sensitized Rh-negative mothers had Rh-negative newborns, yet these mothers had increases in the anti-D titer during pregnancy.[20,21]

Amniotic Fluid Spectrophotometry

In 1961, Liley advocated amniotic fluid spectrophotometry for more accurately determining severity in HDN.[23] A composite graph indicating three zones correlating with mild, intermediate and high risk for severe HDN was established according to gestational age (Fig 7-1). The OD450 measured in a sample of amniotic fluid obtained during the third trimester is used to determine the Δ OD 450 (ie, the deviation from linearity at 450 nm, the absorption spectrum of bilirubin). Read-

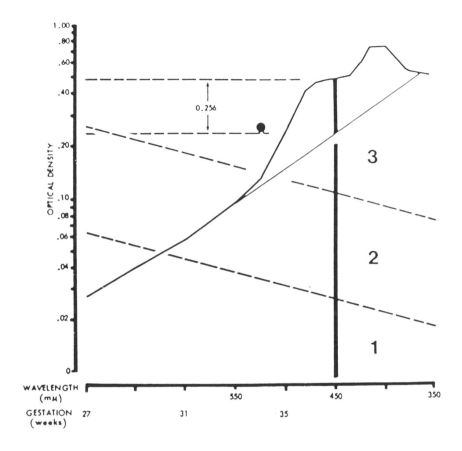

Figure 7-1. Amniotic fluid optical density rise at 450 nm 0.256 (Zone 3) is shown; a further rise at 405-410 nm indicates either oxyhemoglobin from contaminating blood or heme secondary to severe hemolysis. This fetus was delivered early at 34.5 weeks and was prehydropic, requiring four exchange transfusions. (Used with permission from Bowman JM, Pollock JM.[17])

ings in zone 3 indicate that severe disease and hydrops are present or will develop in a few days. Zone 1 readings indicate probably no disease is present, but there is still a 10% chance of the neonate requiring exchange transfusion. Zone 2 readings indicate a moderate risk of the disease becoming more severe as the zone 3 boundary is approached. The overall accuracy of prediction of HDN severity is 95%,[12] but this can only be achieved with serial Δ OD 450 measurements. The accuracy of prediction is much better in the third trimester than in the second trimester, and caution must be used when extrapolating the zones to earlier than 28 weeks of gestation.[24]

Although the incidence of traumatic amniocentesis has decreased significantly with the advent of ultrasonic guidance, there remains a 2% risk of this complication.[25] If it occurs, placental hemorrhage results in blood in the amniotic fluid, producing 580-, 540- and 415-nm oxyhemoglobin peaks that obscure the 450-nm peak. In addition, placental hemorrhage may further immunize the mother with fetal blood increasing the severity of HDN.

Ultrasonography

Ultrasonography has significantly improved the antenatal management of HDN since its development in the 1970's.[26] Fluid accumulations, such as ascites and enlarged organ size, seen in the hydropic fetus can be determined using this technique. Moreover, the location of the placenta and fetal vessels can be determined, allowing safer amniocentesis, umbilical cord sampling and transfusion procedures. In intraperitoneal and direct intravascular transfusion, the presence of blood in the fetal peritoneal cavity or turbulence in the umbilical vessels can be confirmed.

Ultrasound studies are limited in that only overt hydrops can be detected, as ultrasonography is not able to detect impending hydrops. Fetuses can become severely anemic, with hematocrits less than 0.10 (10%) in some cases without manifesting hydrops fetalis.[11] Therefore, reliance on ultrasonography alone to monitor disease severity may result in the failure to detect severely anemic, nonhydropic fetuses. However, others experienced with using ultrasonography in the monitoring of HDN find it a valuable tool in the detection of fetal distress prior to the development of overt hydrops.

Percutaneous Umbilical Blood Sampling

Advanced generations of ultrasound equipment in the 1980's allowed the obstetrician to safely access the fetal circulation using PUBS. This, in turn, provided another major enhancement in the antenatal management of HDN. Fetal blood sampling (FBS) is now recognized as the most accurate way of determining the degree of severity of fetal hemolytic disease in the absence of hydrops. When performed on fetuses without platelet or coagulation abnormalities, the procedure is relatively safe, with a reported fetal mortality of less than 1%.[27] One drawback is that FBS does result in a high incidence of fetomaternal hemorrhage, and therefore should only be undertaken in the context of HDN when: 1) amniotic fluid Δ OD 450 rises into the upper 75% level of zone 2, 2) when an anterior placenta cannot be avoided at amniocentesis or 3) maternal pregnancy history and/or maternal alloantibody titers place the fetus at risk. A fourth possible indication is the situation in which the father is heterozygous for the offending antigen and the previous infant(s) have been severely affected. In this case, FBS should be used for determining fetal blood type with respect to the incompatible antigen, as well as for measuring other parameters of hemolysis.

FBS can be performed as early as 18 weeks of gestation and is generally feasible by 20 weeks. The safest sampling site is at the insertion of the umbilical vein in the placenta.

Suppression of Maternal Alloimmunization

A number of therapies have been utilized in attempts to suppress the immune response to fetal red cell antigens in mothers who are already immunized. Rh hapten,[28] Rh-positive red cell stroma[29] and administration of RhIG[30] (in contrast to its success in Rh HDN prevention) have all been shown to be ineffective in reversing or suppressing an established immune response to Rh. Only two approaches have resulted in the suppression of established immunity: 1) plasmapheresis of the mother[31,32] and, more recently, 2) intravenous immune globulin (IVIG) infusions to the mother.[33]

For plasma exchange, a protocol of exchanging 10-20 liters weekly, replacing with albumin-saline solution and supplementing with IVIG, may reduce the antibody levels as much as 75%. However, after several weeks of such therapy, antibody levels may rebound.[12] Other investigators contend that small volume plasmapheresis (0.6 L/wk) results in decreases in anti-D titers and can obviate the need for intrauterine transfusion in some cases.[34] It is reasonable to consider this therapy if one is treating a very severely affected fetus early in gestation (prior to 20 weeks) as a temporizing measure until the fetus is of an adequate size to receive intrauterine transfusions (22-24 weeks). Some recommend that plasmapheresis be used only for mothers with histories of having hydropic fetuses at or before 24-26 weeks of gestation and whose husbands are homozygous for the offending antigen. Intensive plasmapheresis should begin at 10-12 weeks when transfer of maternal IgG is beginning. Amniocentesis or FBS should be done at around 18 weeks of gestation in such cases.

IVIG may ameliorate fetal hemolysis in severely alloimmunized women.[33] A recent report of IVIG in Rh alloimmunization found that in 24 patients receiving 0.4 g/kg for 4-5 days every 2-3 weeks until delivery, there was a significant decrease in anti-D titers and intrauterine hemolysis after treatment was instituted. No adverse effects were reported on mothers of fetuses attributed to IVIG. The best results were obtained if IVIG was started before 28 weeks on nonhydropic fetuses.[35] Maternal alloantibody levels decrease after IVIG doses of 2 g/kg. It is unclear how IVIG may effect this benefit. The immune globulin may nonspecifically block Fc receptors in the placenta involved in transfer of maternal antibody or the fetal reticuloendothelial system from ingesting IgG-coated cells. The administration of IVIG should occur at the same time in gestation as is recommended for aggressive plasmapheresis. Doses of 0.4 to 1.0 g/kg maternal body weight for 5 or 2 days, respectively, should be given at 2-6 week intervals. Amniotic fluid and/or FBS at 18-20 weeks should not be omitted if the mother is receiving IVIG.

Despite reports of success with plasmapheresis and IVIG given to the mother, these therapies may fail entirely or be only partially effective, in which case intrauterine transfusion may still be necessary.

Management of the Fetus

The main challenge since 1945 has been the reduction of fetal mortality and morbidity due to HDN. Early delivery was shown in the early 1950's to reduce fetal deaths due to HDN, since the neonate who was destined to become hydropic at 32-34 weeks could be treated with exchange transfusions ex-utero. However, the tradeoff was significant morbidity and mortality due to prematurity.[36] Despite this, by 1961, the perinatal mortality for HDN was reduced from 25% to under 20%.[12]

Intrauterine transfusion of the fetus has allowed otherwise severely affected fetuses to remain in utero longer in order to reduce the risks of prematurity and to address HDN. This is particularly helpful for the 8% of HDN fetuses who become hydropic prior to 31 weeks of gestation.

Intraperitoneal transfusion (IPT) was demonstrated to be effective in 1963.[37] Red cells placed in the fetal peritoneal cavity will gradually be adsorbed into the fetal circulation over a few days and will function normally. Diaphragmatic movement is necessary for this absorption and, therefore, if the fetus is apneic, no adsorption will occur. The absorption is somewhat less efficient when edema is present. IPT has resulted in an overall salvage rate in severely affected fetuses of 76%.[12]

Drawbacks of IPT include its lack of efficacy in the nonbreathing, hydropic fetus; the difficulty encountered when the placenta is anterior, leading to increased traumatic fetal deaths; and the high rate (30%) of spontaneous labor induction.[12]

Many of these difficulties were addressed with the development of direct intravascular fetal transfusion (IVT). Initially, IVT was done through the fetoscope; however, an extremely high degree of skill is required of the operator, as visualization of important structures to be targeted and avoided is poor. The advances in ultrasound (see above) allowed FBS as well as IVT in the umbilical vein at lower risk than intraperitoneal techniques or IVT through the fetoscope.

Under ultrasound guidance, the tip of a 20-22 gauge spinal needle is introduced into an umbilical blood vessel, preferably the vein, at its insertion into the placenta. When the needle tip appears to be in the appropriate vessel, as assessed by ultrasound, blood is withdrawn and determination of fetal source is made by rapid alkaline denaturation test, by serologic red cell typing with anti-I or other pertinent marker[38] or by red cell size (MCV). Once the location of the needle tip in the fetal vessel is confirmed, gamma irradiated packed red cells [hematocrit of 0.75-0.80 (75-80%)] are infused at a dose of about 50 mL/kg estimated nonhydropic fetal weight.[12,38] Direct IVT does not rely upon diaphragmatic movement to be effective and, therefore, this technique can salvage even moribund, hydropic, nonbreathing fetuses.

There are two situations in which IPT may still be superior to IVT: when the placenta is posterior and the insertion of the fetal vessels into the placenta is not accessible to the IVT needle, and when the fetal vessels are abnormally small and will not accommodate the transfusion needle.[12]

Management of the Neonate

The use of exchange transfusions in severely affected neonates reduced the perinatal mortality from 50% to 25%.[12] Still other therapies, including phototherapy, phenobarbital and albumin infusion, have reduced the need for exchange transfusions. Today, postnatal measurements of free bilirubin and other indices of hemolysis can identify with precision which neonates will benefit from exchange transfusion and which do not need them.

Prevention of Maternal Alloimmunization

Perhaps the most exciting chapter in the HDN story is the success of RhIG prophylaxis for mothers at risk of alloimmunization during pregnancy. The routine administration of RhIG to Rh-negative mothers at 28 weeks of gestation (and again 12 weeks later, if the mother has not delivered) is recommended. A postpartum dose is not given if delivery occurs within 3 weeks of the second dose; otherwise, it should be given within 72 hours of delivery. The postpartum dose should be augmented if there was significant (greater than 25 mL) fetomaternal hemorrhage, according to the estimate of total fetal cells in the maternal circulation. In addition, prophylaxis should be given after spontaneous and therapeutic abortions, amniocenteses and fetal blood sampling.

The history, mechanism of action and current recommendations for RhIG prophylaxis were recently included in an AABB publication and the reader is referred to this excellent review for further information.[12]

Neonatal Alloimmune Thrombocytopenic Purpura

Neonatal alloimmune thrombocytopenic purpura (NATP) manifests before or shortly after birth and is caused by maternal alloimmunization to a paternal (fetal) platelet antigen not present on the mother's platelets. The incidence of alloimmune thrombocytopenia in the fetus and neonate is about 1 in 2000 live births.[39]

Pathophysiology

The mechanism of platelet destruction in NATP is analogous to that of the red blood cell destruction in HDN. Expression of the immunizing antigen on fetal platelets, eg, Pl^{A1}, occurs by 19 weeks of gestation.[40] Transplacental passage of the antigen may occur even earlier. In turn, maternal IgG is produced, crosses the placenta, coats fetal platelets and ultimately causes their destruction.

Although there is a similar pathogenesis of NATP and HDN, NATP is distinguished from the latter by a high rate of affected first pregnancies, up to nearly 60% of cases occurring in primiparae.[41] Therefore, immunization of mothers to platelet antigens must occur more readily than to the usual red cell antigens implicated in HDN.

The antigen most commonly implicated in this disease is Pl^{A1} (HPA-1a), a platelet-specific antigen located on glycoprotein IIIa. Incompatibility for Pl^{A1} is found in 46-83% of all cases.[42-45] Its allele, Pl^{A2} (HPA-1b), has also been linked to NATP.[46,47] Other platelet-specific alloantigens involved in NATP are Bak (HPA-3),[48,49] Pen(Yuk) (HPA-4),[50,51] Br (HPA-5),[39,52] Ko (HPA-2)[53,54] and Ca (Tu) (HPA-6).[55] Antibodies to HLA Class I antigens are thought to be causative in a few cases[56] although a true association between HLA antibodies, which are quite common in pregnancy, and fetal or neonatal thrombocytopenia is unproven.

The existence of an incompatibility for a platelet antigen between mother and fetus appears to be necessary, but insufficient for maternal immunization to occur. Since 98% of the Caucasian population is positive for the Pl^{A1} antigen, fetuses of 2% of women are at risk for developing NATP. However, far fewer than 2% of normal pregnancies are affected by this disorder. The lower than expected rate of NATP does not appear to be due to under-reporting, since prospective and retrospective studies of pregnancies arrive at about the same incidence.[57] It is probable that a specific immune response gene(s) is (are) required in order for a Pl^{A1}-negative mother to produce anti-Pl^{A1}. Indeed, there are several studies describing significant associations between anti-Pl^{A1} production and specific HLA phenotypes.[58-62] To date, the strongest link appears to be with the DR52a allele found in nearly 100% of $Pl^{A2/A2}$ mothers who produce anti-Pl^{A1}.[63]

The severity of NATP is quite variable, some patients demonstrating only mild thrombocytopenia without bleeding and others presenting with evidence of extensive in-utero intracranial hemorrhage (ICH). A number of factors may be related to the severity of NATP.

Although never rigorously studied, the specificity of the antiplatelet antibody may correlate with severity of NATP. It appears that the most severe cases, those within in-utero ICH for instance, are most often related to incompatibilities for Pl^{A1}. Anti-Pen^a, although a less commonly implicated antibody in NATP, has also been reported to cause in-utero ICH. Similarly, Bak^a and Pl^{A2} have been linked to severe NATP with perinatal ICH. To date, ICH has not been reported to occur in anti-Br^a-mediated NATP, despite Br^a being the second most commonly implicated antigen, after Pl^{A1}, in this disease.[39]

The apparent differences in severity of NATP, according to the antigen involved, may relate to the density of target molecules on fetal platelets. The most densely represented antigen systems on the platelet surface are Pl^A and Pen, both found on glycoprotein IIIa (GPIIIa), with approximately 20,000 sites each per platelet in the heterozygous, affected fetus. Ten thousand to 15,000 Bak sites (located on GPIIb) are on each heterozygous platelet. In contrast, Br^a or Br^b, located on GPIa/IIa, are present at only 1000-2000 sites per platelet. This may explain why the more severe cases of NATP have incompatibilities for Pl^A, Pen or Bak system antigens.

If antigen density is related to disease severity, one would expect antigen density to be inversely related to platelet count in the affected fetus. This has not been adequately studied to date, but there are at least three cases of severe fetal thrombocytopenia [$<10 \times 10^9$/L ($<10,000/\mu$L) platelets] in NATP related to Br system antigens.[39,64] Therefore, severe NATP, although less likely when a "low density" antigen is implicated, cannot be ruled out on that basis alone. As in HDN, in NATP there is some evidence that birth order is related to severity. Although not as well studied as in HDN, subsequent pregnancies in NATP are at least as severely affected as, if not more so than, the initially affected pregnancy in a family.[65] There are exceptions in that a few cases have been reported in which subsequent pregnancies seem to be less severely affected than the first. Such factors as early delivery by cesarean section and having platelet support readily available for subsequent deliveries are confounding variables that affect the severity of subsequent births.

The nature of the maternal antibody has been examined as a possible factor contributing to the severity of the disease. Prenatal serum testing of the mother is useful in predicting severity in some cases,[42,49,66-68] but is not always reliable.[69,70] In one series,[70] 25 pregnancies were monitored with prenatal maternal serum testing. While the presence of a platelet-specific antibody prenatally predicted neonatal thrombocytopenia (Table 7-2), the severity of thrombocytopenia could not ade-

Table 7-2. Birth Platelet Counts According to Presence or Absence of Maternal Platelet Antibodies*

	Yes	No	p Value
Presence of any antibody	69,954 (n = 22)	43,500 (n = 2)	NS
Presence of platelet-specific antibody	31,250 (n = 16)	138,750 (n = 8)	<0.005
Presence of anti-Pl^{A1}	34,285 (n = 14)	243,000 (n = 2)	<0.001

*Twenty-five women who were at risk for delivering infants with NATP were followed prospectively using three anti-platelet antibody assays (platelet suspension immunofluorescence test, ^{51}Cr release and antigen capture ELISA). Mean cord blood or birth platelet counts in the infants were correlated with presence of any platelet-reactive antibody (including anti-HLA) and with platelet-specific antibody, including anti-Pl^{A1}.[70]

quately be predicted by the changes in antibody titer throughout pregnancy (Table 7-3). A more recent study of maternal antibody characteristics found a correlation between the ability of the antibody to fix complement, the titer of anti-Pl^{A1} and the occurrence of fetal or neonatal ICH.[71] Of interest, these serologic findings were more closely associated with the risk of ICH than was the platelet count in the fetus.

Table 7-3. Changes in Antibody Strength Throughout Pregnancy

Patient Number	Platelet Antibody Tests*			Neonatal Platelet Count (per μL)
	PSIFT	^{51}Cr Release	ACE	
5	Increase	Negative	Stable	7,000
6	Decrease	Decrease		35,000
8	Increase	Increase	Stable	18,000
9	Increase	Negative	Decrease	27,000
13†	Decrease	Increase	Decrease	16,000; 21,000
16	Negative	Negative	Decrease	31,000
17	Decrease	Negative	Decrease	83,000
19	Decrease	Negative		19,000
20	Decrease	Increase		60,000
25	Decrease	Decrease	Decrease	41,000
26	Negative	Stable		54,000

*Increases or decreases in antibody strength did not correlate with the severity of neonatal thrombocytopenia.[70]
†This Pl^{A1}-negative woman delivered twins.
PSIFT = Platelet suspension immunofluorescence test.
ACE = Antigen-capture enzyme-linked immunosorbent assay.

Clinical Features

As many as 81% of affected infants have petechiae, purpura or overt bleeding at birth.[42] Since approximately half of the cases occur in first pregnancies, many of these infants are delivered vaginally, hence bleeding symptoms may be associated with forceps trauma or cephalohematomas. By one estimate, 28% have evidence of central nervous system hemorrhage diagnosed in the neonatal period.[42]

Up to one half of the ICHs occur prenatally.[72,73] These intrauterine intracranial hemorrhages in NAT are characterized by severe neurologic sequelae, porencephaly and optic hypoplasia.[74] In-utero ICH is particularly worrisome because it cannot be avoided by elective cesarean section. Formerly thought to occur only between 30 and 35 weeks of gestation, in-utero ICH is now recognized to occur as early as 13 weeks of gestation.[75,76] An additional complication of NATP is late-onset neurologic deficits that are not noted clinically in the neonatal period.[77]

If untreated, the thrombocytopenia in NATP normally lasts 2-3 weeks and then resolves spontaneously. There are cases, however, in which the thrombocytopenia is unusually prolonged.[48,54]

Laboratory Diagnosis

Neonatal platelet counts are uniformly low and hemoglobin concentrations are occasionally decreased secondary to bleeding. After 72-96 hours, the serum bilirubin may be elevated due to passive resorption of extravasated blood. A bone marrow aspirate is occasionally performed to determine the source of severe thrombocytopenia, and megakaryocytes are usually present in normal numbers. In at least three cases, however, decreased megakaryocytes were reported.[54,78,79]

If NATP is suspected on the basis of clinical and routine laboratory studies, platelet antibody studies can confirm the diagnosis. Platelet antigen typing of the parents is used to detect relevant platelet antigen incompatibilities. Screening of the maternal serum for platelet-specific antibodies demonstrates an antibody of the expected specificity in 85% of cases.[45,80]

A variety of platelet antibody assays have been used for platelet typing and to detect platelet-reactive antibodies in maternal serum. These include: indirect immunofluorescence, chromium-51 release, complement fixation, platelet agglutination and mixed passive hemagglutination. More recently, enzyme-linked immunosorbent assays (ELISA)that test the mother's serum against immobilized platelet glycoprotein targets have been used for the detection and identification of NATP antibodies.[55,64,69,70,81] These methods appear promising in that they exclude interfering HLA antibodies and more clearly delineate the presence of platelet-specific alloantibodies.

Differential Diagnosis

Clinical diagnosis of NATP requires that infection and other causes of fetal/neonatal thrombocytopenia be excluded. Blood cultures and serum antivirus titers are usually required to exclude the possibility of either bacterial or viral infection. Disseminated intravascular coagulation related to either infection or to another underlying cause can be diagnosed with routinely available coagulation tests. Maternal autoimmune thrombocytopenia is an important cause of neonatal thrombocytopenia. A careful maternal history regarding possible past history of thrombocytopenia as well as a current maternal platelet count are necessary to exclude the possibility of a maternal autoantibody causing fetal thrombocytopenia. Other more unusual causes of neonatal thrombocytopenia should also be considered. These include drug exposure in the mother (particularly to quinine, quinidine or thiazides), hemangioma thrombocytopenia syndrome, congenital amegakaryocytic hypoplasia, thrombocytopenia with absent radius (TAR) syndrome, congenital leukemia, histiocytosis and Wiscott-Aldrich syndrome. These other causes of NATP can generally be excluded by a physical examination, by a careful maternal history for drug exposure and by routine laboratory studies.

Prognosis

The prognosis of NATP is generally good. The reported overall mortality is between 6.5 and 14%.[42,43,82] ICH occurs in between 15 and 28% of all cases reported,[41,58,82] and up to one-half of these intracranial events may occur prenatally.[72,73]

Second and subsequent siblings often have a better prognosis than first affected children, probably due to preventive measures such as elective cesarean deliveries and immediate compatible platelet transfusions, which are not available to their older siblings.[42] The most difficult obstacle in reducing morbidity and mortality from this disease is the fact that most cases continue to be diagnosed retrospectively, with a low neonatal platelet count or severe hemorrhage being the first sign of fetal platelet destruction. Until and unless prenatal screening options designed to detect a potentially affected fetus are available to all pregnant women, this will continue to be the case.

Antenatal Management

In contrast to HDN, there are no screening programs in place for detecting mothers at risk of delivering infants affected with NATP. Therefore, in most cases, no antenatal management is possible. However, in subsequent pregnancies or in pregnancies in sisters of affected mothers, there is an opportunity to detect affected fetuses and plan appropriate perinatal care or administer antenatal therapy if necessary. As in HDN, the management of subsequent pregnancies at risk for NATP relies on several tools.

Maternal History

A history of delivering a thrombocytopenic infant in the past is an important clue in determining the risk of NATP in subsequent pregnancies. Such a history must be carefully researched to determine: 1) that other causes of neonatal thrombocytopenia were excluded; 2) that the mother's platelet count during the previous pregnancy was normal (to exclude maternal autoimmune thrombocytopenia); 3) that responses to platelet transfusions or other therapy were consistent with alloimmune thrombocytopenia; and 4) that any platelet serology evaluation was compatible with NATP (see below).

Identifying the Implicated Antigen

If a serologic diagnosis was made after the previous affected pregnancy, this will serve as a guide to the management of the current pregnancy. The prediction of second and subsequent siblings being affected is aided by the knowledge of gene frequencies of the antigen systems involved (Table 7-4). In the case of Pl^{A1}, the gene frequency data predict that about 87% of subsequent pregnancies will be affected, ie, would have the relevant antigen incompatibility. In a series reported by Shulman, 97% of second and subsequent pregnancies were actually affected.[41] This suggests that there is probably a reporting bias, with subsequent affected infants more often reported than unaffected infants.

Paternal Zygosity Testing

The prediction that a particular fetus carries the incompatible antigen can be aided by determining the zygosity of the father. Most recognized platelet-specific alloantigens occur in diallelic systems. Therefore, all fathers of fetuses at risk are either homozygous for the offending antigen, or heterozygous for it, his other allele being the other member of the alloantigenic system. For zygosity testing, the father's platelets are typed for both alleles of the implicated antigen system. For instance, in a case of NATP due to anti-Pl^{A1}, the father's platelets can be typed for Pl^{A1} and Pl^{A2} to categorize him as either homozygous or heterozygous for the gene that determines Pl^{A1} antigen status. If he is a heterozygote, there is approximately a 50% chance that he will pass the Pl^{A1} gene to a subsequent offspring, resulting in an affected neonate. Alternately, a homozygous Pl^{A1} father almost certainly will pass the incompatible antigen to the fetus. In the event the father's platelets possess a double dose of the implicated antigen, there is no need to determine the platelet type of the fetus, as it will be an obligate heterozygote.

Fetal Genotyping

Whereas prediction of an affected fetus with a father homozygous for the offending antigen is relatively simple, ie, all such offspring will

Table 7-4. Human Platelet Alloantigen System*

Alloantigen System	Allelic Forms	Phenotypic Frequency		Risk of Subsequent[†] Affected Fetus According to Maternal Antibody Specificity	
Pl^A (HPA-1)	Pl^{A1} (HPA-1a)	72%	$Pl^{A1/1}$	Anti-Pl^{A1}	86.75%
		26%	$Pl^{A1/2}$		
	Pl^{A2} (HPA-1b)	2%	$Pl^{A2/2}$	Anti-Pl^{A2}	53.60%
Ko (HPA-2)	Ko^b (HPA-2a)	85%	$Ko^{b/b}$	Anti-Ko^b	92.14%
		14%	$Ko^{a/b}$		
	Ko^a (HPA-2b)	1%	$Ko^{a/a}$	Anti-Ko^a	53.35%
Bak (HPA-3)	Bak^a (HPA-3a)	37%	$Bak^{a/a}$	Anti-Bak^a	71.7%
		48%	$Bak^{a/b}$		
	Bak^b (HPA-3b)	15%	$Bak^{b/b}$	Anti-Bak^b	61.9%
Pen (HPA-4)	Pen^a (HPA-4a)	99%	$Pen^{a/a}$	Anti-Pen^a	>99%
		<0.1%	$Pen^{a/b}$		
	Pen^b (HPA-4b)	<0.1%	$Pen^{b/b}$	Anti-Pen^b	~50%
Br (HPA-5)	Br^b (HPA-5a)	80%	$Br^{b/b}$	Anti-Br^b	89.7%
		19%	$Br^{a/b}$		
	Br^a (HPA-5b)	1%	$Br^{a/a}$	Anti-Br^a	52.5%

*Phenotypic frequencies for the platelet antigen systems shown are for the Caucasian population only. Significant differences in gene frequencies may be found in African and Asian populations.
†Assuming a first-affected pregnancy has been diagnosed with NATP and an incompatibility with the expected antibody was found on parental typing and maternal serum screen. This estimate also assumes the father was not typed for the alternate allele.

inherit the incompatible antigen, determining the risk of an affected fetus with a heterozygous father can be difficult. Obtaining a fetal blood sample for determination of fetal platelet type carries with it the inherent risk of the sampling procedure, which, if the fetus is thrombocytopenic, may be significant (see later). Moreover, the sample obtained may not be adequate for standard serologic platelet typing methods. Recently, the discovery of the genetic polymorphisms associated with the allelic differences in the Pl^{A},[83] Bak,[84] Pen,[85] Ko[86] and Br (Newman PJ, personal communication) alloantigen systems allows the determination of fetal genotypes for these antigen systems. With as little as 1 mL of fetal blood or 5-10 mL of amniotic fluid, the platelet alloantigen genotypes for these systems can be determined using allele-specific oligonucleotide probes of polymerase chain reaction (PCR)- amplified fetal genomic DNA.[68] This technique allows early detection of affected second and subsequent fetuses so that prenatal treatment can be considered, if appropriate.

Fetal Ultrasound

Whereas fetal ultrasound is still helpful in the management of HDN fetuses, in that ascites and hydrops can be detected, signaling the need for in-utero intervention with fetal transfusions, this technology is not particularly helpful in preventing damage to the fetus in NATP. It is possible to obtain fetal ultrasound studies prior to delivery to detect gross central nervous system damage due to ICH. Cranial ultrasound examination may reveal sonolucent areas in the brain or intraventricular hemorrhage. Often, fetal ultrasound detects old ICHs that are cystic. Once ICH is detected, the damage is often irreversible.

Percutaneous Umbilical Blood Sampling

PUBS allows clinicians to assess fetal platelet count early in pregnancy. As early as 18 weeks of gestation, PUBS can be performed on a pregnancy at risk to obtain fetal platelets for counting and/or platelet antigen typing.[65,87,88] If early PUBS indicates that the fetus is affected, subsequent PUBS can be done to monitor prenatal therapy in the mother. Currently, maternal IVIG with or without steroid therapy is under study for cases at high risk of severe thrombocytopenia and in-utero ICH.[89] Another application of PUBS is the quantifying of fetal platelets, together with transfusion of maternal platelets (or other antigen-negative platelets) to the fetus during the pregnancy.[72,90-93] This latter approach is a heroic intervention and is best reserved for those pregnancies at extreme risk for in-utero ICH.

Fetal Scalp Vein Sampling

When PUBS is not available, the fetal platelet count may be assessed using fetal scalp vein sampling before committing to a vaginal delivery. In general, a platelet count $>50 \times 10^9/L$ ($>50,000/\mu L$) indicates that a vaginal delivery can proceed without undue risk. However, a platelet count $<50 \times 10^9/L$ ($<50,000/\mu L$) indicates that the infant should be delivered by cesarean section. The use of fetal scalp vein sampling does not address the problem of ICH, which has been reported to occur as early as 13 weeks of gestation.[75] An additional problem associated with fetal scalp vein sampling is that the platelet count on the sample may be falsely low, leading to unnecessary cesarean deliveries.[94]

Management of Maternal Alloimmunization

Once NATP is diagnosed in a family, in subsequent pregnancies, one is faced with the alloimmunized mother whose immune system is already primed to respond to the fetus carrying the incompatible platelet antigen. As yet, there are no viable approaches for the prevention of platelet antigen alloimmunization and, therefore, prenatal therapies have been directed at attempting to blunt an established immune response. Since second or subsequent affected fetuses in a family are rarely, if ever, less severely affected than the first affected child, prenatal intervention to reduce the mother's immune response is rational. PUBS should be considered as early as 18-20 weeks of gestation to document fetal platelet count and to obtain fetal blood to establish the fetal platelet type if necessary, depending on the paternal zygosity. Alternatively, if determination of the fetal platelet genotype is required, this can be done even earlier in pregnancy using the lower risk amniocentesis[69] (16-17 weeks) or chorionic villus sampling[75] (8-12 weeks) to obtain fetal cells for DNA-based typing.

If thrombocytopenia is present, maternal IVIG treatment can be given in weekly doses of 1 g/kg until delivery. Approximately 4-5 weeks after IVIG therapy is begun, a repeat PUBS should be considered to assess treatment success. If there has been no response, dexamethasone is added, according to one ongoing clinical trial. Although these studies are still in progress, it appears that, overall, a 75% response rate to maternal IVIG with or without corticosteroids might be expected in such pregnancies.[89] It is still too early to assess the benefit of adding steroids to the IVIG therapy, but the current clinical trial should answer this question.

In the initial seven patients treated antenatally with IVIG reported by Bussel et al, six responded with increasing or stabilizing fetal platelet counts, and none of the seven neonates suffered ICH. This was in contrast to three of their previously affected siblings.[65] Drawbacks of the therapy included possible oligohydramnios and small-for-gestational-age infants that may have been related to the IVIG or steroids used in the trial. A follow-up experience was reported by the same group with 18 mothers receiving IVIG prenatally.[95] Each of the 18 had had at least one severely affected child with NATP. Forty-eight percent of these children had had ICH, six occurring in utero. The median fetal platelet count increased by about 100% [32×10^9/L to 60×10^9/L (32,000/µL to 60,000/µL] and none of the treated infants had ICH. A comparison was made to the birth platelet count of the previous affected siblings (Fig 7-2).

Three patients failed therapy in this study. In one, the platelet count never increased above 6×10^9/L (6000/µL) and the fetus was given an in-utero platelet transfusion and was delivered by elective cesarean section. The second patient was the only woman in the series whose gamma globulin was administered in a dose of less than 1 g/kg/wk. The third was receiving IVIG and steroids. Despite the lack of response in the platelet count of these three infants, no ICH occurred.

In the subsequent randomized trial, in which mothers were randomized to receive IVIG alone or in combination with dexamethasone, no complications have been detected that could be related to the

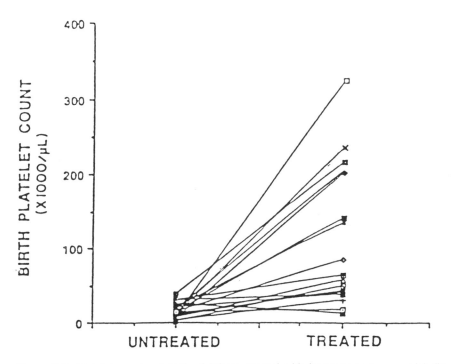

Figure 7-2. Platelet counts at birth of infants treated with intravenous gamma globulin compared with those of their untreated siblings. (Used with permission from Lynch L et al.[95])

drugs. However, a total of eight fetuses were lost after the initial PUBS procedure attempting to qualify for either the pilot studies or the randomized trial. The risk was most apparent in fetuses with very low [<10×10^9/L (<10,000/µL)] cord blood platelet counts.

This complication led to the recent recommendation that all initial and follow-up cord sampling on potentially thrombocytopenic fetuses be performed followed by rapid infusion of compatible platelets. The platelets can be harvested from the mother or other compatible platelet donor in a double manual plateletpheresis procedure or a shortened machine plateletpheresis procedure. The platelets must be washed free of maternal serum in AB plasma or saline, irradiated with gamma irradiation (30 Gy is recommended), concentrated to a volume of 10-15 mL and given to the obstetrician performing the PUBS. If there is delay in obtaining machine or manual platelet counts on the fetal samples, it is reasonable to infuse these platelets even before the fetal platelet count is available. The small risk of infusing platelets in a fetus with a normal platelet count is outweighed by the benefit of preventing fetal exsanguination through the PUBS puncture site while the platelet count is awaited.

One potential problem identified with harvesting maternal platelets after antenatal IVIG therapy has been initiated is that infectious disease markers in maternal serum may become positive due to passive antibody in the IVIG preparation. Because of this possibility, a pre-IVIG serum sample should be obtained and reserved for infectious disease markers testing in the event that maternal platelets are required for fetal or neonatal transfusion.

Additional trials of high dose IVIG therapy as antenatal treatment have had mixed results. Kaplan et al[91] and Mir et al [96] failed to prevent fetal thrombocytopenia in their patients treated before the 35th week of gestation with 0.4 g/kg/day for 5 days and 0.8 g/kg followed by 0.4 g/kg/week, respectively. However, Bussel et al were successful in managing seven pregnant women using IVIG at a dose of 1.0 g/kg/wk for 6-17 weeks prior to delivery.[65,91,96] It was postulated by Lynch[95] and later by Shwe et al[97] that the higher dose of IVIG given beginning early in the third trimester may be important in achieving a therapeutic threshold to ameliorate the fetal thrombocytopenia. The latter reported a recent case of a woman with a history of two previously affected infants, one with ICH, who underwent IVIG therapy beginning at 35 weeks of gestation in the third pregnancy. The dose given was 0.4 g/kg/day for 3 days and then 0.4 g/kg/day for 1 day in weeks 36 and 37. Elective cesarean section was performed at 38 weeks and a normal infant was delivered with a platelet count of 161×10^9/L (161,000/µL.) He was confirmed to be Pl^{A1} positive, incompatible with the maternal antibody. This case points up the variability in responses to IVIG. The mechanism of action in reducing the severity of NATP is not understood. Hypotheses include blockade of placental or fetal Fc receptors and immune modulation of the mother's alloantibody.

Steroids are not generally considered to be adequate as sole therapy to ameliorate maternal platelet alloimmunization; however, one case report by Daffos et al appeared to contradict this conventional wisdom. A severely affected fetus with a platelet count of only $20 \times 100/L$ (20,000/µL) at 23 weeks was treated via the mother receiving oral prednisolone, 10 mg daily. The platelet count in the fetus was observed to increase over the next 12 weeks and at delivery was $80 \times 10^9/L$ (80,000/µL). The authors comment that such a rise in platelet count has not been reported to occur spontaneously and suggest that this moderate dose of steroids may have been responsible for the positive response.[98]

Management of the Affected Fetus

An alternative approach is to give the fetus repeated transfusions of antigen-negative platelets either immediately before delivery[91] or at weekly intervals beginning at 18-20 weeks and continuing throughout the pregnancy.[72,92,93] This treatment is more complex than its counterpart in HDN where the survival of transfused compatible RBCs can be expected to be about 3 weeks. In the case of transfused platelets, 5-7 days is about the maximum survival that can be anticipated (Fig 7-3). This then obligates the mother to receive weekly intrauterine platelet transfusions to maintain safe levels of fetal platelets. The platelets must be volume-reduced and washed if they are derived from the mother (approximately 0.4×10^{11} in 5-10 mL) and gamma-irradiated prior to infusion to the fetus. In one very interesting recent report, a mother who was alloimmunized to both Pl^{A1} and HLA antigens had had three fetal losses due to ICH at progressively earlier time points in gestation (28, 19 and 16 weeks). The last of these pregnancies had been managed with maternal IVIG without success. In the fourth pregnancy, weekly intraperitoneal injections of IVIG were given to the fetus in utero until 18 weeks. It is unclear if this was successful, as the fetal platelet count at 18 weeks was only 12 $\times 10^9/L$ (12,000/µL) and a pretreatment platelet count was not obtainable. The fetus was then given Pl^{A1}-negative platelets from an allogeneic donor. The authors concluded that these platelets had unexpectedly short survival because of the anti-HLA antibodies present in the mother. The fetus was then transfused with maternal platelets that had much better survival. Ultimately, a normal infant was delivered after 20 in-utero platelet transfusions. The authors state that this is the first report of HLA antibodies complicating in-utero platelet transfusion in NATP.[99]

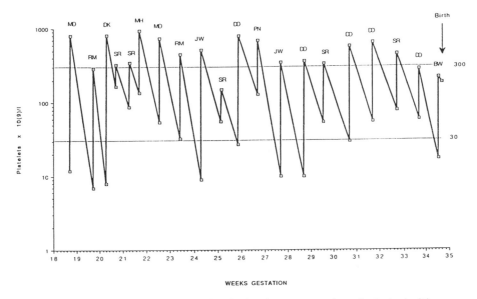

Figure 7-3. Fetal platelet transfusions during the fourth pregnancy of a patient who had three severely affected fetuses in the past. Pretransfusion and posttransfusion fetal platelet counts are shown. The authors distinguish between the platelet survival of transfusions from donor SR, the mother and other PI^{A1}-negative donors who were not compatible with the mother's HLA antibodies. (Used with permission from Murphy MF et al.[99])

Management of an Affected Neonate

The major treatment goal in NATP is to increase the neonate's platelet count. In a severely thrombocytopenic neonate [<20-30 × 10⁹/L (<20,000-30,000/µL), a platelet transfusion should be given. Platelets compatible with the maternal antibody are ideal since they will not be destroyed by passive antibody in the neonate's serum.[42,100] The most readily available source of such platelets is usually the mother. However, transfusing maternal plasma along with maternal platelets may prolong the course of neonatal thrombocytopenia. It is necessary, therefore, to remove maternal plasma and resuspend the platelets in either normal AB plasma or normal saline.[101,102] Alternative donors of compatible platelets may be found among the mother's siblings or in some cases regional blood centers have files of donors known to be negative for the antigens implicated in NATP.

Maternal platelets are usually provided as soon as possible after the diagnosis of NATP is made in the first affected neonate in a family. In second or subsequent pregnancies, cesarean section is recommended to prevent birth trauma. The maternal platelets can be obtained the day before planned delivery. In a unique modification of maternal platelet transfusion, one institution obtained maternal platelets 3 months prior to expected delivery and cryopreserved them. Maternal platelets frozen in dimethyl sulfoxide were then available immediately after birth. This approach prevented the mother from having to donate platelets shortly before cesarean section.[103]

If maternal or other antigen-negative platelets are not readily available and the neonate is in urgent need of a transfusion, random donor platelet transfusions should not be withheld. Responses to random donor platelets may be adequate, albeit temporary, and therefore emergent use of these products is warranted in severely affected neonates if compatible platelets are not on hand.

A newer approach to the treatment of NATP is the use of high-dose IVIG, usually at a dose of 0.4 g/kg/day for 5 days. Reports to date show variable responses. The platelet count usually increases within the first 24-48 hours; however, in some cases up to 8 days are required for the platelet count to begin to increase.[104-106] The slow rate of response compared to that achieved with compatible platelet transfusion, in which the response is immediate, argues that the use of IVIG as a sole therapy for NATP should be avoided if there is a serious risk of thrombocytopenic hemorrhage. The mechanism of action of IVIG in this disorder is unknown. It is possible that either reticuloendothelial cell blockade prevents antibody-coated platelets from being consumed or that the antibodies in the IVIG interfere with the interaction of maternal antiplatelet-antibody with fetal platelets (anti-idiotypic antibodies).

References

1. Diamond LK, Blackfan KD, Baty JM. Erythroblastosis fetalis and its association with universal edema of the fetus, icterus gravis neonatorum and anemia of the newborn. J Pediatr 1932; 1:269-309.
2. Levine P, Stetson RE. An unusual case of intra-group agglutination. JAMA 1939;113:126-7.
3. Landsteiner K, Wiener AS. An agglutinable factor in human blood recognized by immune sera for rhesus blood. Proc Soc Exp Biol Med 1940;43:223.
4. Levine P, Katzin EM, Burnham L. Isoimmunization in pregnancy: Its possible bearing on the etiology of erythroblastosis fetalis. JAMA 1941;116:825-7.
5. Mollison PL, Engelfriet CP, Contreras M. Blood transfusion in clinical medicine. 9th ed. London: Blackwell Scientific Publications, 1993.

6. Chown B. Anemia from bleeding of the fetus into the mother's circulation. Lancet 1954;1:1213-15.

7. Kleihauer E, Braun H, Betke K. Demonstration von fetalem Haemoglobin in den Erythrozyten eines Blutausstriches. Klin Wochenschr 1957;35:637-8.

8. Bowman JM, Pollock JM, Penston LE. Fetomaternal transplacental hemorrhage, during pregnancy and after delivery. Vox Sang 1986;51:117-21.

9. Bowman JM. Hemolytic disease of the newborn. Can Med Asoc J 1974;111:318.

10. Yeung CY, Hobbs JR. Serum-gamma-G-globulin levels in normal premature, post-mature, and "small for dates" newborn babies. Lancet 1968;1:1167-70.

11. Frigoletto FD, Greene JF, Benacerraf BR, et al. Ultrasonographic fetal surveillance in the management of the isoimmunized pregnancy. N Engl J Med 1986;315:430-2.

12. Bowman JM. Historical overview: Hemolytic disease of the fetus and newborn. In: Kennedy MS, Wilson SM, Kelton, JG, eds. Perinatal transfusion medicine. Arlington, VA: American Association of Blood Banks, 1990:1-52.

13. Gemke RJBJ, Kanhai HHH, Overbeeke MAM, et al. ABO and rhesus phenotype of fetal erythrocytes in the first trimester of pregnancy. Br J Haematol 1986;64:689-97.

14. Kanhai HHH, Gravenhorst J, van't Veer MB, et al. Chorionic biopsy in management of severe rhesus isoimmunization. Lancet 1984;2:157-8.

15. Kanhai HH, Gravenhorst J, Gemke RJ, et al. Fetal blood group determination in first trimester pregnancy for the management of severe immunization. Am J Obstet Gynecol 1987;156;120-3.

16. Bowell PJ, Selinger M, Ferguson J, et al. Antenatal fetal blood sampling for the management of alloimmunized pregnancies: Effect upon maternal anti-D potency levels. Br J Obstet Gynaecol 1988;95:759-64.

17. Bowman JM, Pollock JM. Amniotic fluid spectrophotometry and early delivery in the management of erythroblastosis fetalis. Pediatrics 1965;35:815-35.

18. Judd WJ, Luban NLC, Ness PM, et al. Prenatal and perinatal immunohematology: Recommendations for serologic management of the fetus, newborn infant, and obstetric patient. Transfusion 1990;30:175-83.

19. Bowell PJ, Wainscot JS, Peto TEA, Gunson HH. Maternal anti-D concentrations and outcome in rhesus haemolytic disease of the newborn. Br Med J 1982;285:327-9.

20. Nance SJ, Nelson JM, Horenstein J, et al. Monocyte monolayer assay: An efficient noninvasive technique for predicting the

severity of haemolytic disease of the newborn. Am J Clin Pathol 1989;92:89-92.

21. Urbaniak SJ, Greiss MA, Crawford RJ, Fergusson MJC. Prediction of the outcome of rhesus haemolytic disease of the newborn: Additional information using an ADCC assay. Vox Sang 1984;46:323-9.

22. Brouwers HAA, Overbeeke MAM, Ertbruggen, et al. What is the best predictor of the severity of ABO-haemolytic disease of the newborn? Lancet 1988;2:641-4.

23. Liley AW. Liquor amnii analysis in management of pregnancy complicated by rhesus immunization. Am J Obstet Gynecol 1961;82:1259-71.

24. Ananth U, Queenan JG. Does midtrimester Δ OD 450 of amniotic fluid reflect severity of Rh disease? Am J Obstet Gynecol 1989;161:47-9.

25. Bowman JM, Pollock JM. Transplacental fetal hemorrhage after amniocentesis. Obstet Gynecol 1985;66:749-54.

26. Chitkara U, Wilkins I, Lynch L, et al. The role of sonography in assessing severity of fetal anemia in Rh- and Kell-isoimmunized pregnancies. Obstet Gynecol 1988;71:393-8.

27. Daffos F, Capella-Pavlovsky M, Forestier F. Fetal blood sampling during pregnancy with use of a needle guided by ultrasound: A study of 6067 consecutive cases. Am J Obstet Gynecol 1985;153:655-60.

28. Carter BB. Preliminary report on a substance which inhibits anti-Rh serum. Am J Clin Pathol 1947;17:646-9.

29. Gold WR Jr, Queenan JT, Woody J, et al. Oral desensitization in Rh disease. Am J Obstet Gynecol 1983;146:980-1.

30. De Silva M, Contreras M, Mollison PL. Failure of passively administered anti-Rh to prevent secondary Rh immune responses. Vox Sang 1985;48:178-80.

31. Graham-Pole J, Barr W, Willoughby MLN. Continuous flow plasmapheresis in management of severe Rhesus disease. Br Med J 1977;1:1185-8.

32. Robinson EAE, Tovey LAD. Intensive plasma exchange in the management of severe Rh disease. Br J Haematol 1980;45:621-31.

33. de la Camara C, Arrieta R, Gonzalez A, et al. High dose intravenous immunoglobulin as the sole prenatal treatment for severe Rh immunization. N Engl J Med 1988;318:519-20.

34. Bennebroek-Grauenhorst J. Management of serious alloimmunization in pregnancy. Vox Sang 1988;55:1-8.

35. Margulies M, Voto L, Mathet E, Margulies M. High dose intravenous IgG for the treatment of severe Rhesus alloimmunization. Vox Sang 1991;61:181-9.

36. Chown B, Bowman WD. The place of early delivery in the prevention of foetal death from erythroblastosis. Pediatr Clin North Am 1958;May:279-85.

37. Liley AW. Intrauterine transfusion of fetus of haemolytic disease. Br Med J 1963;2:1107-9.

38. Steiner EA, Judd WJ, Oberman HA, et al. Percutaneous umbilical blood sampling and umbilical vein transfusions. Transfusion 1990;30:104-8.

39. Mueller-Eckhardt C, Kiefel V, Grubert A, et al. Immunological and clinical evaluation of 348 cases of suspected neonatal alloimmune thrombocytopenia. Lancet 1989;1:363-6.

40. Kaplan C, Patereau C, Reznikoff-Etievant MF, et al. Antenatal Pl^{A1} typing and detection of GPIIb-IIIa complex. Br J Haematol 1984;60:586.

41. Shulman NR, Jordan JV. Platelet immunology. In: Coleman RW, Hirsh J, Marder VJ, Salzman EW, eds. Hemostasis and thrombosis. Philadelphia: JB Lippincott, 1987:452-529.

42. Deaver JE, Leppert PC, Zaroulis CG. Neonatal alloimmune thrombocytopenic purpura. Am J Perinatol 1986;3:127-31.

43. Pearson HA, Shulman NR, Marder VJ, Cone TE Jr. Isoimmune neonatal thrombocytopenic purpura: Clinical and therapeutic considerations. Blood 1964;23:154-77.

44. Shulman NR, Jordan JV. Platelet immunology. In: Coleman RW, Hirsch J, Marder VJ, Salzman EW, eds. Hemostasis and thrombosis. Philadelphia: JB Lippincott, 1982;274-342.

45. von dem Borne AEGKr, van Leeuwen EF, von Riesz LE, et al. Neonatal alloimmune thrombocytopenia: Detection and characterization of the responsible antibodies by the platelet immunofluorescence test. Blood 1981;57:649-56.

46. Mueller-Eckhardt C, Becker T, Weisheit M, et al. Neonatal alloimmune thrombocytopenia due to fetomaternal Zw^b incompatibility. Vox Sang 1986;50:94-6.

47. Maslanka K, Lucas GF, Gronkowska A, et al. A second case of neonatal alloimmune thrombocytopenia associated with anti-Pl^{A2} (Zw^b) antibodies. Haematologia (Budap) 1989;22:109-13.

48. Miller DT, Etzel RA, McFarland JG, et al. Prolonged neonatal alloimmune thrombocytopenic purpura associated with anti-Bak(a): Two cases in siblings. Am J Perinatol 1987;4:55-8 [see erratum Am J Perinatol 1987;4:177].

49. von dem Borne AEGKr, von Riesz E, Verheugt FWA, et al. Bak^a, a new platelet-specific antigen involved in neonatal alloimmune thrombocytopenia. Vox Sang 1980;39:113-20.

50. Friedman JM, Aster RH. Neonatal alloimmune thrombocytopenic purpura and congenital porencephaly in two siblings associated with a "new" maternal antiplatelet antibody. Blood 1985;65:1412-5.

51. Shibata Y, Matsuda I, Miyaji T, Ichikawa Y. Yuk^a, a new platelet antigen involved in two cases of neonatal alloimmune thrombocytopenia. Vox Sang 1986;50:177-80.
52. Kiefel V, Santoso S, Katzmann B, et al. A new platelet specific alloantigen Br^a. Vox Sang 1988;54:101-6.
53. Shulman NR, Marder VJ, Hiller MC, Collier EM. Platelet and leukocyte isoantigens and their antibodies: Serologic, physiologic and clinical studies. Prog Hematol 1964;4:222-304.
54. Bizzaro N, Dianese G. Neonatal alloimmune amegakaryocytosis. Vox Sang 1988;54:112-4.
55. McFarland JG, Blanchette V, Collins J, et al. Neonatal alloimmune thrombocytopenia due to a new platelet-specific alloantibody. Blood 1993 (in press).
56. Sternbach MS, Malette M, Nadon F, Guevin RM. Severe alloimmune neonatal thrombocytopenia due to specific HLA antibodies. Curr Stud Hematol Blood Transfus 1986;52:97-103.
57. Blanchette VS, Chen L, Salomon de Friedberg Z, et al. Alloimmunization to the Pl^{A1} platelet antigen: Results of a prospective study. Br J Haematol 1990;74:209-15.
58. Mueller-Eckhardt C, Mueller-Eckhardt G, Willen-Ohff H, et al. Immunogenicity of and immune response to the human platelet antigen Zwa is strongly associated with HLA-B8 and DR3. Tissue Antigens 1985;26:71-6.
59. Reznikoff-Etievant MF, Muller JY, Kaplan C, et al. L'immunisation contre l'antigène plaquettaire Zw^a (Pl^{A1}): Groupe à risque, prévention des complications. Pathol Biol 1986;34:783-7.
60. Reznikoff-Etievant MF, Dangu C, Lobet R. HLA-B8 antigen and anti-Pl^{A1} allo-immunization. Tissue Antigens 1981;18:66-8.
61. DeWaal LP, van Dalen CM, Engelfriet CP, von dem Borne AEGKr. Alloimmunization against the platelet specific Zw^a antigen, resulting in neonatal alloimmune thrombocytopenia or posttransfusion purpura is associated with the supertypic DRw52 antigen including DR3 and Drw6. Hum Immunol 1986;17:45-53.
62. Mueller-Eckhardt G, Mueller-Eckhardt C. Alloimmunization against the platelet specific Zw^a antigen associated with HLA-DRw52 and/or DRw6? Hum Immunol 1987;18:181-2.
63. Valentin N, Vergracht A, Bignon JD, et al. HLA-DRw52a is involved in alloimmunization against Pl^{A1} antigen. Hum Immunol 1990;27:73.
64. Kiefel V, Shechter Y, Atias D, et al. Neonatal alloimmune thrombocytopenia due to anti-Brb (HPA-5a). Vox Sang 1991;60:244-5.
65. Bussel J, Berkowitz R, McFarland J, et al. Antenatal treatment of neonatal alloimmune thrombocytopenia. N Engl J Med 1988; 319:1374-8.

66. Deaver JE, Leppert PC, Zaroulis CG. Neonatal alloimmune thrombocytopenic purpura: A case report. Am J Obstet Gynecol 1986;154:153-5.
67. Sia CG, Amigo NC, Harper RG, et al. Failure of cesarean section to prevent intracranial hemorrhage in siblings with isoimmune neonatal thrombocytopenia. Am J Obstet Gynecol 1985;153:79-81.
68. Naido S, Messmore H, Caserta V, Fine M. CNS lesions in neonatal isoimmune thrombocytopenia. Arch Neurol 1983;40:552-4.
69. McFarland JG, Aster RH, Bussel JB, et al. Prenatal diagnosis of neonatal alloimmune thrombocytopenia using allele-specific oligonucleotide probes. Blood 1991;78:2276-82.
70. McFarland JG, Frenzke M, Aster RH. Testing of maternal sera in pregnancies at risk for neonatal alloimmune thrombocytopenia. Transfusion 1989;29:123-33.
71. Bussel JB, McFarland JG, NAIT Working Party. The chromium release assay correlates with intracranial hemorrhage in neonatal alloimmune thrombocytopenia. Pediatric Research 1990;27:139.
72. Waters A, Murphy M, Hambley H, Nicolaides K. Management of alloimmune thrombocytopenia in the fetus and neonate. In Nance SJ, ed: Clinical and basic science aspects of immunohematology. Arlington, VA: American Association of Blood Banks, 1991:155-177.
73. Neonatal immune thrombocytopenia working party. Neonatal alloimmune thrombocytopenia (NAIT): Information derived from a prospective international registry (abstract). Pediatr Res 1986;23:337a.
74. Davidson JE, McWilliam RC, Evans TJ, Stephenson JBP. Porencephaly and optic hypoplasia in neonatal isoimmune thrombocytopenia. Arch Dis Child 1989;64:858-60.
75. Johnson JM, McFarland JG, Blanchette VS, et al. Prenatal diagnosis of neonatal alloimmune thrombocytopenia using an allele-specific oligonucleotide probe. J Prenatal Diagnosis 1993 (in press).
76. Giovangrandi Y, Daffos F, Kaplan C, et al. Very early intracranial hemorrhage in alloimmune fetal thrombocytopenia. Lancet 1990;336:310.
77. Sitarz AL, Driscoll JM, Wolff JA. Management of isoimmune neonatal thrombocytopenia. Am J Obstet Gynecol 1976;124:39-42.
78. Adner MM, Fisch GR, Starobin SG, Aster RH. Use of "compatible" platelet transfusions in treatment of congenital isoimmune thrombocytopenic purpura. N Engl J Med 1969;280:244-7.
79. Pearson HA, McIntosh S. Neonatal thrombocytopenia. Clin Haematol 1978;7:111-22.
80. Mueller-Eckhardt C, Kayser W, Forster C, et al. Improved assay for detection of platelet specific Pl^{A1} antibodies in neonatal alloimmune thrombocytopenia. Vox Sang 1982;43:76-81.

81. Kiefel V, Santoso S, Mueller-Eckhardt C. A new platelet-specific alloantigen Br^a. Vox Sang 1988;54:101-6.

82. Kaplan C, Daffos F, Forestier F, et al. Current trends in neonatal alloimmune thrombocytopenia: Diagnosis and therapy. In: Kaplanj-Gouet C, Schlegel N, Salmon Ch, McGregor J, eds. Platelet immunology: Fundamental and clinical aspects. Paris: Colloque INSERM/John Liffey Erotext, 1991:267.

83. Newman PJ, Derbes RS, Aster RH. The human platelet alloantigens, Pl^{A1} and Pl^{A2}, are associated with a leucine33/proline33 amino acid polymorphism in membrane glycoprotein IIIa, and are distinguishable by DNA typing. J Clin Invest 1989;83:1778-81.

84. Lyman S, Aster RH, Visentin GP, Newman PJ. Polymorphism of the human platelet membrane glycoprotein IIvb associated with the Bak^a/Bak^b alloantigen system. Blood 1990;75:2343-8.

85. Wang R, Furihata K, McFarland JG, et al. An amino acid polymorphism within the RGD binding domain of platelet membrane glycoprotein IIIa is responsible for the formation of the Pen^a/Pen^b alloantigen system. J Clin Invest 1992;90:2038-43.

86. Kuijpers RW, Faber NM, Cuypers HT, et al. NH2-terminal globular domain of human platelet glycoprotein Ib alpha has a methionine 145/threonine 145 amino acid polymorphism, which is associated with the HPA-2 (Ko) alloantigens. J Clin Invest 1992;89:381-4.

87. Daffos F, Forestier F, Muller JY, et al. In utero platelet transfusion in alloimmune thrombocytopenia. Lancet 1984;2:1103-4.

88. Reznikoff-Etievant MF. Management of alloimmune neonatal and antenatal thrombocytopenia. Vox Sang 1988;55:193-201.

89. Bussel JB, McFarland JG, Lynch L, et al. Antenatal treatment of alloimmune thrombocytopenia (abstract). Blood 1991;78:1540a.

90. Daffos F, Forestier F, Muller JY, et al. Prenatal treatment of alloimmune thrombocytopenia (letter). Lancet 1984;2:632.

91. Kaplan C, Daffos F, Forestier F, et al. Management of alloimmune thrombocytopenia: Antenatal diagnosis and in utero transfusion of maternal platelets. Blood 1988;72:340-3.

92. Nicolini U, Rodeck CH, Koshenour NK, et al. In utero platelet transfusion for alloimmune thrombocytopenia (letter). Lancet 1988;2:506.

93. Murphy MF, Pullon HWH, Metcalfe P, et al. Management of fetal alloimmune thrombocytopenia by weekly in utero platelet transfusions. Vox Sang 1990;58:45-9.

94. Christiaens GCML, Helmerhorst FM. Validity of intrapartum diagnosis of fetal thrombocytopenia. Am J Obstet Gynecol 1987; 157:864-5.

95. Lynch L, Bussel JB, McFarland JG, et al. Antenatal treatment of alloimmune thrombocytopenia. Obstet Gynecol 1992;80:67-71.

96. Mir N, Samson D, House MJ, Kovar IZ. Failure of antenatal high dose immunoglobulin to improve fetal platelet count in neonatal alloimmune thrombocytopenia. Vox Sang 1988;55:188-9.

97. Shwe KH, Love EM, Lieverman BA, Newland AC. High dose intravenous immunoglobulin in the prenatal management of neonatal alloimmune thrombocytopenia. Clin Lab Haematol 1991;13:75-9.

98. Daffos F, Forestier F, Kaplan C. Prenatal treatment of fetal alloimmune thrombocytopenia (letter). Lancet 1988;2:910.

99. Murphy MF, Metcalf P, Waters AH, et al. Antenatal management of severe feto-maternal alloimmune thrombocytopenia: HLA incompatibility may affect responses to fetal platelet transfusions. Blood 1993;81:2174-9.

100. Katz J, Hodder FS, Aster RS, et al. Neonatal isoimmune thrombocytopenia: The natural course and management and the detection of maternal antibody. Clin Pediatr 1984;23:159-62.

101. Mennuti M, Schwartz RH, Gill F. Obstetric management of isoimmune thrombocytopenia. Am J Obstet Gynecol 1974;118: 565-6.

102. Vesilind GW, Simpson MB, Shifman MA, et al. Evaluation of a centrifugal blood cell processor for washing platelet concentrates. Transfusion 1988;28:46-51.

103. McGill M, Mayhaus C, Hoff R, Carey P. Frozen maternal platelets for neonatal thrombocytopenia. Transfusion 1987;27:347-9.

104. Suarez CR, Anderson C. High dose intravenous gammaglobulin (IVG) in neonatal immune thrombocytopenia. Am J Hematol 1987;26:247-53.

105. Derycke M, Dreyfus M, Ropert JC, Tchernia G. Intravenous immunoglobulin for neonatal isoimmune thrombocytopenia. Arch Dis Child 1985;60:667-9.

106. Sidiropoulos D, Straume B. The treatment of neonatal isoimmune thrombocytopenia with intravenous immunoglobin (IgG IV). Blut 1984;48:383-6.

In: Nance ST, ed.
Alloimmunity: 1993 and Beyond
Bethesda, MD: American Association of Blood Banks, 1993

8

Prospects for Modulation of Alloimmunity

David D. Eckels, PhD

A LLOIMMUNITY IS A RECENTLY understood phenomenon that has perplexed immunologists and frustrated transplant surgeons for more than 30 years. To understand current prospects for controlling or modulating alloimmunity, the different immune molecules that are involved must first be appreciated at the structural level. This chapter will present the phenomenon of alloimmunity, the various molecular structures involved, the consequences of alloimmune recognition and, finally, the ways in which alloimmunity might be modulated.

Alloimmunity

Alloimmunity is distinguished from "regular" immunity based on its specificity for allogeneic tissues. As will be shown later, this distinction is somewhat artificial, but it illustrates the intimate relationship between alloimmunity and transplantation. Sir Peter Medawar first described the laws of transplantation: *Isografts are accepted; allografts are rejected.* His initial observations of graft acceptance and rejection in animal models arose from the underlying phenomenon of alloimmune recognition and he probably provided a major contribution to the rationale for studying the organismal, cellular and molecular basis of alloimmunity.[1] As the idea was dawning that organ transplantation between unrelated individuals might be possible, it was also clear that something had to be done to overcome the "second" law of transplan-

David D. Eckels, PhD, Senior Investigator, Immunogenetics Research Section, The Blood Center of Southeastern Wisconsin, Milwaukee, Wisconsin
(This work is supported by Research Career Development Award AI00799 and grants AI22832 and HL44612 of the Blood Research Foundation.)

tation by finding ways to block the alloimmune process by which transplants were rejected.

Fairly early on, it was discovered that a variety of agents could inhibit immunologic responses, including alloimmunity. Drugs, originally used in cancer chemotherapy because of their ability to kill or inhibit rapidly dividing cells, were also found to suppress lymphocytes that must divide in order to respond to antigens, and with variable results, similarly impeded allograft rejection.[2] Cytotoxic antibodies targeted to the cells of the immune system were also effective at inhibiting graft rejection and some are in use today, for example, antilymphocyte globulin (ALG). The major problem with ALG and various drugs, as well as similar agents, is that they nonspecifically suppress the immune system. Therefore, while they may block allograft rejection, they also block all other immunologic responses nonspecifically and render the recipient susceptible to a variety of life-threatening viral and microbial infections. Many of these may represent normal flora that are usually kept at bay with a healthy immune system. In view of the dire consequences of compromised immunologic responses, it has been the goal of many scientists to develop ways of blocking *antigen-specific* immune responses such that, for example, responses to allografted tissue are inhibited, but those to infectious agents are left intact. The accomplishment of this aim would require a detailed understanding of the complete physiology of the rejection process and would also lead to profound insights into the workings of the normal immune system.

A Digression

Normal immune recognition is said to be "self" restricted. This is based on a series of observations, made by Shevach and Rosenthal[3,4] and later by Zinkernagel and Doherty,[5] that are worth understanding in order to appreciate the prospects for modulating alloimmunity. Taking advantage of the fact that lymphocytes divide rapidly upon encountering antigen, radioactive labeling of newly synthesized DNA provides an index of immunologic response *in vitro*, which can be used to dissect some of the requirements of immune recognition. T lymphocytes, isolated from strain 2 guinea pigs, were found to respond to antigen only when that antigen was presented by macrophages from the same strain. Similarly, strain 13 T lymphocytes would only respond to antigen when it was presented by strain 13 macrophages, but not by strain 2 antigen-presenting cells (APCs). This phenomenon was termed self-restriction because only "self" APCs were able to present antigens to "self" T cells. Furthermore, it was found to be controlled by genes of the major histocompatibility complex (MHC) and thus T-cell recognition is also said to be MHC-restricted. This phenomenon was dissected further by taking advantage of inbred mouse strains that were congenic for genes of the MHC and would thus allow genetic mapping of self- or MHC-restricted recognition. As in the experiments above, T lymphocytes recognized viral antigens only when presented by APC with matching MHC genes. An unexpected development of this work was the observation that different kinds of immunologic responses were restricted by different classes of MHC genes. Thus, proliferative responses were restricted by MHC Class II molecules whereas cytotoxicity, killing of virus-infected target cells, was restricted by MHC Class I molecules.

The "Paradox" of Alloimmunity

Given that T cells are normally self-restricted, it is puzzling that they should also be able to recognize allogeneic MHC molecules or transplantation antigens. Furthermore, it is also clear that recognition of allogeneic Class II molecules leads to proliferation and amplification of alloimmune responses, whereas alloantigen-specific killer cells recognize allogeneic Class I molecules on transplanted tissue. In the absence of precise structural information, it was difficult to understand what seemed like a paradox. How is it that T cells come to recognize allogeneic MHC molecules when they seem to be programmed to recognize antigens associated with self MHC proteins? This conundrum is exacerbated by our understanding of developmental immunology wherein T cells undergo what is known as positive selection in that they must interact successfully with self MHC molecules in the thymus in order to emerge as fully competent peripheral T lymphocytes. Thus, responsiveness to foreign antigens also involves a re-encounter with self MHC molecules; how could allogeneic MHC molecules be recognized if T cells could never have been exposed to them during thymic ontogeny? Part of the answer to these questions is provided by a structural understanding of the molecules involved in both self-restricted and allo-restricted T-cell recognition. Recent crystallographic evidence and molecular genetic analysis of the genes encoding immune recognition structures now provide important insights into the mysteries of T-cell specificity.

Structure of the MHC and Encoded Molecules

The MHC of humans is called the HLA system and spans approximately 4 megabases on the short arm of chromosome 6.[6] Despite this length, MHC genes are most often inherited as a unit, called a haplotype, probably because of evolutionary pressure to keep together genes involved in common functions. An emerging observation is that the MHC encodes genes that are involved in the processing and presentation of antigens that can be recognized by T lymphocytes. In the HLA system, this includes genes for Class I, Class II, complement, transporter, proteasome, heat-shock, collagen, tumor necrosis factor and other molecules, including those of unknown function. Much is known about the Class I and Class II genes because they encode the histocompatibility or transplantation antigens. They come in a large variety of allelic forms and thus are polymorphic. This polymorphism not only is allelic, but also is present at the haplotype level in that different haplotypes may have different numbers of loci. It is this extraordinary diversity, almost unique in any given individual, that frustrates transplant surgeons and fascinates immunogeneticists.

The Class I and Class II genes are structurally different. Class I genes are composed of the HLA-A, -B, -C, -E, -F, -G and -H loci, in addition to a number of pseudogenes, all of which have probably arisen through a process of gene duplication. Class I genes are composed of eight exons and encode a single molecule of 44 kD. Class I allelic variation may run into the hundreds for HLA-B, but HLA-A and -C also vary extensively. Class II genes encode an α chain of approximately 33 kD and a β chain of around 28 kD within five and six exons, respectively. These are organized into three major series, HLA-DR, -DQ and -DP and two genes of minor importance, DOB and DNA. Class II DRB genes vary in number with respect to the various haplotypes, thereby extending the level of polymorphism even further. Unlike the DP and the DQA genes, the DRA gene is essentially nonpolymorphic. Other Class II sequences are variably expressed with obscure functions, but are evidence of extensive gene duplication within the Class II region. Minimal estimates of Class II allelic diversity include 26 alleles for DP, at least 20 for DQ and more than 75 for DR. Polymorphism at the DNA level is directly transcribed and translated into polymorphism at the protein level. The extent to which such diversity is immunologically significant has not been fully elucidated. However, clues are provided by analysis of MHC protein structures and it is reasonable to presume that even single amino acid differences have measurable impact on immune function.[7]

HLA molecules come in two forms. Class I molecules form heterodimers with the 12 kD β$_2$-microglobulin and are expressed at the surface of all cells as glycosylated transmembrane proteins or in soluble form in the serum. Only the Class I heavy chain spans the membrane and has been shown to be involved in intracellular signaling.[8,9] The importance of soluble HLA molecules is unknown. Class II molecules also consist of α and β chain heterodimers, although both are encoded within the MHC. Both are also glycosylated transmembrane proteins. Class II molecules have also been shown recently to be involved in transmembrane signaling.[10-14] Both Class I and Class II molecules are members of what is known as the immunoglobulin gene superfamily, which is composed of proteins with a characteristic domain structure wherein 50-60 amino acid, disulfide-bounded loops are assembled together as molecular subunits; each domain corresponds to a particular exon. The crystallographic structure of Class I and Class II molecules is also known and both are remarkably similar.[15-17] Each has two membrane-proximal, immunoglobulin-like domains on top of which is found a platform of eight anti-parallel β-sheets over which arch two parallel α-helices. Between the α-helices is a deep groove that has been shown to bind small peptide fragments of antigens (Fig 8-1). It is this *complex* of MHC and peptide that is recognized by T cells.[18]

The structural information on MHC molecules has led to important insights into immune recognition. Consistent with the phenomenon of MHC restriction, T cells probably interact with both peptide antigen and the α-helical regions of the MHC molecule. Thus, peptides are recognized in the "context" of the Class I or Class II molecule. Further-more, the context of T-cell recognition has important functional con-sequences for the T cell in that helper, CD4 T cells recognize exogenous

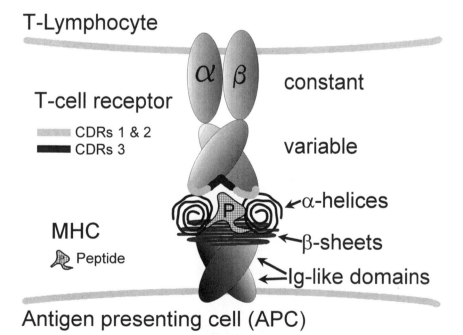

T-Lymphocyte

T-cell receptor

CDRs 1 & 2
CDRs 3

α β

constant

variable

←α-helices

←β-sheets

←Ig-like domains

MHC

Peptide

Antigen presenting cell (APC)

Figure 8-1. The trimolecular complex. Peptide is presented on the MHC platform and recognized by the T-cell receptor. Specificity for peptide and MHC elements is dictated (hypothetically) by contact regions on the immunoglobulin-like receptor, complementarity determining region (CDR) 3 of both the TCR α and β chains for peptide and CDRs 1 and 2 for MHC. This trimolecular interaction forms the basis of T-cell recognition and subsequent activation. (© David D. Eckels, 1993. Used with permission.)

foreign peptides bound to Class II molecules, whereas cytotoxic, CD8 T cells recognize internally derived peptide antigens bound to the groove of Class I molecules. It is also quite clear that MHC molecules are capable of binding an immense array of peptides and that this array probably varies based on the allelic polymorphism that is largely confined to the internal surfaces of the antigen-binding groove. Thus, depending on the side chains of amino acids that form the internal surface of the groove, peptide binding and conformation will be variously affected depending on the local side-chain chemistry. This concept is of great significance with respect to alloimmunity because the peptides will probably be derived from fairly ubiquitous proteins leading to different or similar peptide derivatives that will probably bind in conformations different from those induced by binding to self MHC molecules. Consistent with this hypothesis, observations have been made that T cells may recognize peptides derived from MHC molecules, serum albumin or other conserved proteins.[19,20] It is also clear that the surface of the MHC molecule that provides for T-cell contact is relatively well-conserved because most of the polymorphism lies within the peptide binding groove.

Therefore, the paradoxical aspects of alloimmune recognition are dissipated with the realization that alloimmunity involves "self"-restricted recognition of different peptide derivatives or conformational variants of autologous proteins if "self" is used to mean the conserved face or surface of the MHC molecule.[21] Additionally, alloimmune recognition can involve processing of alloantigens by autologous antigen-presenting cells such that peptide derivatives of allogeneic MHC antigens are presented in association with self MHC molecules to self-restricted T cells. Thus, alloimmunity involves two mechanisms of recognition, either or both of which may lead to allograft rejection or graft vs host disease (GVHD). Based on animal models, this is likely to involve a two-step process whereby differences in allogeneic Class II molecules are recognized by CD4 helper cells that amplify the immune response through the production of various lymphokines and induce the differentiation of allospecific cytolytic precursor cells into the mature CD8 killer cells that are probably ultimately responsible for graft destruction. Although beyond the scope of this treatment, the potential role of other inflammatory cells in alloimmune responses should not be overlooked.

Potentials for Modulating Alloimmunity

The tripartite structure involved in alloimmune recognition provides at least three points of antigen-specific intervention. These include interference with recognition at the level of the MHC, the T-cell receptor and the peptide. In addition, recent studies have shown that it may be possible to take advantage of secondary signaling requirements in unexpected ways that may yet produce the desired effect of inhibiting alloantigen-specific responses (Fig 8-2).

MHC Molecules

Both in-vitro and in-vivo studies have adequately demonstrated that antibodies to MHC molecules are able to block T-cell responses effectively. This approach could be useful in cases where a particular antigen is restricted by a specific MHC molecule such as Class I or Class II or their isotypes. For example, let us presume that a bone marrow transplant has been performed with donor and recipient cells that differ at the HLA-B locus and that the recipient is B*2701-positive and the donor is B*2701-negative. Following transplant, GVHD ensues and seems to be directed at the B27 difference. Monoclonal antibodies are available that are specific for B27 antigens and could be used to block the in-vivo response. This approach may be effective when allogeneic molecules themselves are the target of T-cell responses, but it may also be possible to block the afferent phase of immune recognition by antibodies specific for responder MHC mole-

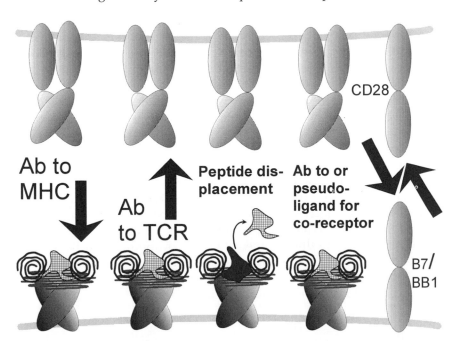

Figure 8-2. Four potential ways to intervene in immunologic responses. 1) Antibody to MHC molecules. 2) Antibody to the T-cell receptor. 3) The use of competitor peptides. 4) Antibody to disrupt signaling through co-receptors. Depending on the circumstances, each of these approaches should enable varying degrees of selective immune modulation. (© David D. Eckels, 1993. Used with permission.)

cules. To extend the B27 example, it is possible that B27-derived peptides are presented in association with donor MHC molecules, which may be restricted to a given Class II isotype or allele of DR, DQ or DP. In this case, isotype- or allele-specific antibodies would be able to block the immune response to the B27 alloantigen while leaving undisturbed the responses restricted by other molecules. Although not qualifying strictly as antigen-specific intervention, this approach does allow for ablation of the relevant responses while leaving the majority of others intact.

T-Cell Receptor

Animal studies have revealed that antigen-specific responses can be blocked by antibodies directed at particular subsets of the T-cell antigen receptor.[22] This is an effective strategy because T-cell responses to individual peptide antigens may be limited to a clonal or oligoclonal population of cells expressing a single T-cell receptor molecule. Obviously, elimination of T cells expressing that particular antigen receptor will eliminate the specific response to cognate antigen. Furthermore, depending on the specificity of the blocking antibody (ie, whether it is T-cell idiotype- or isotype-specific), only a small portion of the T-cell repertoire will be removed. This portion of the repertoire can range from as much as six per 100 T cells if the antibody is specific for a particular $V\beta$ subfamily to one cell in billions if it is idiotype-specific. To the extent that alloimmunity involves the restricted usage of T-cell receptors, this approach will be successful. Evidence that responses to discrete alloantigens involve a limited number of T-cell receptor groups is somewhat contradictory, with in-vitro results generally showing that there is no relationship between the T-cell receptor used and the alloantigen recognized and some in-vivo studies suggesting the opposite. Part of the discrepancy may also have to do with the degree of disparity between responder and stimulator alleles. The modulatory potential of this tactic will not be fully demonstrated until more data are gathered and monoclonal antibodies recognizing very specific groups of T-cell receptor molecules become available. It is noteworthy that the development of such antibodies will be greatly accelerated by the use of transgenic mice that have been tolerized to the framework antigens of human T-cell receptors and hence should respond only to isotypic or idiotypic determinants.[23]

Peptide

Because allorecognition requires particular peptides, substitution of the "wrong" peptides might be able to interfere with alloimmunity. Thus, if an alloresponse is directed at an albumin peptide presented in altered conformation in the context of an allogeneic MHC molecule, then substitution of peptide "X" for albumin should eliminate the particular alloresponse. We have demonstrated just this possibility using T-cell clones specific for allogeneic DRB*0101 molecules and an influenza virus hemagglutinin peptide known to bind to DR1 Class II proteins.[24] Furthermore, to the extent that allorecognition involves processing and presentation of alloantigens by donor cells, it may be possible to provide "competitor" peptides that would effectively block responsiveness. This strategy works quite well when two peptide antigens, known to bind to the same MHC molecule, are provided at the same time in vivo.[25] Perhaps infusion of an allograft with blocking peptides prior to transplantation would lead to enhanced graft survival or minimized GVHD. Especially effective might be the development and use of nonimmunogenic peptides that fail to elicit T-cell responses or through as yet obscure mechanisms may actually be able to render T cells unresponsive or appear to the responding immune system as "self," the donor already being tolerant to such self antigens.

Other Approaches

T-cell activation requires not only binding and signaling through the T-cell receptor, but also the engagement of and activation through other accessory molecules. These include, but are not limited to, CD4, CD8, CD11, CD18 and CD28. As these secondary receptors have been studied, one of their very interesting and important features is that antigen-specific stimulation in the absence of secondary signal seems to result in antigen-specific tolerance. Whereas T cells that have been challenged normally against alloantigens exhibit typical anamnestic responses upon re-exposure to the original antigen, if secondary signaling through CD28, for example, is blocked at the same time that antigen is provided, subsequent rechallenge reveals that the T cells have been rendered specifically unresponsive. The mechanism by which this phenomenon occurs is unknown, but may involve clonal elimination or functional anergy and its advantage is that the immune system's normal capacity for self-regulation is used, perhaps thereby establishing a stable condition of allospecific tolerance. Indeed, two investigators have demonstrated the practicality of this approach. In one, a molecule known as CTLA-4Ig, which is a high-affinity receptor for the CD28 ligand, BB1/B7, has been used to produce specific tolerance in animal models and in human in-vitro studies.[26-28] Another tactic that is poorly understood at the mechanistic level devolves from experiments showing that the presence of T-cell receptor antibodies at the same time as alloantigenic challenge also results in alloantigen-specific unresponsiveness.[29] Therefore, one can envision at the time of transplant, early rather than waiting for rejection episodes to arise, that provision of CTLA-4Ig or anti-T-cell receptor antibody could lead to graft-specific tolerance. Obviously, further testing is required to validate this rationale.

Yet another approach that has not been fully exploited depends upon the route of administration of antigenic stimuli. Although it has long been known that the quality of an immune response often is linked to how antigen is presented (whether orally, intramuscularly, in adjuvant, etc) and allergists and vaccine developers have taken advantage of this knowledge, transplant immunologists have been slow to catch on. One very exciting possibility involves the development of oral tolerance using peptides derived from allogeneic MHC molecules themselves. It seems that simply providing MHC peptides enterically results at least in peptide-specific and perhaps whole antigen-specific tolerance; preliminary evidence is being generated that the acceptance of skin allografts is also extended. Should MHC-specific oral tolerance become workable, it is possible to imagine a pharmacopoeia of peptide "pills" corresponding to all known MHC alleles, the taking of which prior to transplant could precondition the patient toward allograft tolerance!

Summary

Transplantation biology is on the edge of a very exciting era. The maturation of our understanding of immunology at the mechanistic and structural levels should enable us to manipulate the alloimmune response effectively by selective intervention in the sequence of events involving immune recognition, signal transduction and effector responses. It should be noted that this clinical benefit derives from decades of basic work aimed at understanding immunologic mechanisms in both mouse and man. It is hoped that this transmigration of knowledge, from bench to bedside, will continue into the future.

References

1. Eckels DD. Alloreactivity: Allogeneic presentation of endogenous peptide or direct recognition of MHC polymorphism? A review. Tissue Antigens 1990;35:49-55.
2. Waldmann TA. Immune receptors: Targets for therapy of leukemia/lymphoma, autoimmune diseases and for prevention of allograft rejection. Annu Rev Immunol 1992;10:675-704.
3. Rosenthal AS, Shevach EM. Function of macrophages in antigen recognition by guinea pig T lymphocytes. I. Requirements for histocompatible macrophages and lymphocytes. J Exp Med 1973;138:1194-212.

4. Shevach EM, Rosenthal AS. Function of macrophages in antigen recognition by guinea pig T lymphocytes. II. Role of the macrophage in genetic control of the immune response. J Exp Med 1973;138:1213-29.
5. Zinkernagel RM, Doherty PC. MHC-restricted cytotoxic T cells: Studies on the biological role of polymorphic major transplantation antigens determining T cell restriction specificity, function and responsiveness. Adv Immunol 1979;27:51-177.
6. Trowsdale J, Ragoussis J, Campbell RD. Map of the human MHC. Immunol Today 1991;12:443-6.
7. Newton-Nash DK, Eckels DD. Effects of localized HLA class II beta chain polymorphism on binding of antigenic peptide and stimulation of T cells. Hum Immunol 1992;33:213-23.
8. Gilliland LK, Norris NA, Grosmaire LS, et al. Signal transduction in lymphocyte activation through crosslinking of HLA class I molecules. Hum Immunol 1989;25:269-89.
9. Sambhara SR, Miller RG. Programmed cell death of T cells signaled by the T cell receptor and the alpha 3 domain of class I MHC. Science 1991;252:1424-7.
10. Nabavi N, Ghogawala Z, Myer A, et al. Antigen presentation abrogated in cells expressing truncated Ia molecules. J Immunol 1989;142:1444-7.
11. St Pierre Y, Nabavi N, Ghogawala Z, et al. A functional role for signal transduction via the cytoplasmic domains of MHC class II proteins. J Immunol 1989;143:808-12.
12. Cambier JC, Lehmann KR. Ia-mediated signal transduction leads to proliferation of primed B lymphocytes. J Exp Med 1989;170:877-86.
13. Nabavi N, Freeman GJ, Gault A, et al. Signalling through the MHC class II cytoplasmic domain is required for antigen presentation and induces B7 expression. Nature 1992;360:266-8.
14. Kansas GS, Cambier JC, Tedder TF. CD4 binding to major histocompatibility complex class II antigens induces LFA-1-dependent and -independent homotypic adhesion of B lymphocytes. Eur J Immunol 1992;22:147-52.
15. Bjorkman PJ, Saper MA, Samraoui B, Bennett WS, et al. Structure of the human class I histocompatibility antigen, HLA-A2. Nature 1987;329:506-12.
16. Bjorkman PJ, Saper MA, Samraoui B, et al. The foreign antigen binding site and T cell recognition regions of class I histocompatibility antigens. Nature 1987;329:512-18.
17. Brown JH, Jardetzky T, Saper MA, et al. A hypothetical model of the foreign antigen binding site of class II histocompatibility molecules. Nature 1988;332:845-50.
18. Davis MM, Bjorkman PJ. T-cell antigen receptor genes and T-cell recognition. Nature 1988;334:395-402.

19. Rudensky AY, Preston-Hurlburt P, Hong SC, et al. Sequence analysis of peptides bound to MHC class II molecules. Nature 1991;353:622-7.
20. Rudensky AY, Preston-Hurlburt P, al-Ramadi BK, et al. Truncation variants of peptides isolated from MHC class II molecules suggest sequence motifs. Nature 1992;359:429-31.
21. Lombardi G, Sidhu S, Batchelor JR, Lechler RI. Allorecognition of DR1 by T cells from a DR4/DRw13 responder mimics self-restricted recognition of endogenous peptides. Proc Natl Acad Sci USA 1989;86:4190-4.
22. Acha-Orbea H, Mitchell DJ, Timmermann L, et al. Limited heterogeneity of T cell receptors from lymphocytes mediating auto immune encephalomyelitis allows specific immune intervention. Cell 1988;54:263-73.
23. Choi YW, Kotzin B, Lafferty J, et al. A method for production of antibodies to human T-cell receptor beta-chain variable regions. Proc Natl Acad Sci USA 1991;88:8357-61.
24. Eckels DD, Gorski J, Rothbard J, Lamb JR. Peptide-mediated modulation of T-cell allorecognition. Proc Natl Acad Sci USA 1988;85:8191-5.
25. Adorini L, Muller S, Cardinaux F, et al. In vivo competition between self peptides and foreign antigens in T-cell activation. Nature 1988;334:623-5.
26. Linsley PS, Wallace PM, Johnson J, et al. Immunosuppression in vivo by a soluble form of the CTLA-4 T cell activation molecule. Science 1992;257:792-5.
27. Lenschow DJ, Zeng Y, Thistlethwaite JR, et al. Long-term survival of xenogeneic pancreatic islet grafts induced by CTLA4lg. Science 1992;257:789-92.
28. Tan P, Anasetti C, Hansen JA, et al. Induction of alloantigen-specific hyporesponsiveness in human T lymphocytes by blocking interaction of CD28 with its natural ligand B7/BB1. J Exp Med 1993;177:165-73.
29. Anasetti C, Tan P, Hansen JA, Martin PJ. Induction of specific nonresponsiveness in unprimed human T cells by anti-CD3 antibody and alloantigen. J Exp Med 1990;172:1691-700.

Index